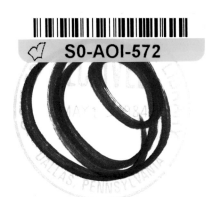

Computers For Medical Office And Patient Management

CTEA

Computers For Medical Office And Patient Management

Edited by

Stacey B. Day, M.D., Ph.D., D.Sc.

Clinical Professor of Medicine, Division of Behavioral Medicine, Department of
Medicine, New York Medical College, Valhalla, New York; Retired Professor of
Biology, Sloan Kettering Division, Cornell University Medical College,
New York; Former Member and Head, Bio-Sciences Communications and
Medical Education, Sloan Kettering Institute for Cancer Research, New York, N.Y.

AND

Jan F. Brandejs, Ph.D.

Formerly Director of Statistics, Systems, and
Economic Research, Canadian
Medical Association, Ottawa, Canada.

VNR VAN NOSTRAND REINHOLD COMPANY
NEW YORK   CINCINNATI   TORONTO   LONDON   MELBOURNE

Manufactured in the United States of America

Published by Van Nostrand Reinhold Company
135 West 50th Street, New York, N.Y. 10020

Van Nostrand Reinhold Limited
1410 Birchmount Road
Scarborough, Ontario M1P 2E7, Canada

Van Nostrand Reinhold Australia Pty. Ltd.
17 Queen Street
Mitcham, Victoria 3132, Australia

Van Nostrand Reinhold Company Limited
Molly Millars Lane
Wokingham, Berkshire, England

15 14 13 12 11 10 9 8 7 6 5 4 3 2 1

Library of Congress Cataloging in Publication Data

Main entry under title:

Computers for medical office and patient management.

 Contents: Introduction to computer-oriented
health informatics / by Stacey B. Day — Doctor's
office computers in the German health system /
by Erhard Geiss — Design principles of computer-
aided physician's office systems / by Jan F.
Brandejs — [etc.]
 1. Medicine—Data processing. 2. Medical offices
—Data processing. I. Day, Stacey B. II. Brandejs,
Jan F. [DNLM: 1. Computers. 2. Practice management,
Medical. W 80 D275c]
R858.C653   610′.28′54   81-11664
ISBN 0-442-21316-6   AACR2

PREFACE

The last 10 years have seen conceptually important advances in the quality of health care. Much of this change is a direct result of the perceptive insights of a small group of physicians dedicated to Health Communications and Biopsychosocial Health.

For the practicing physician dramatic new procedures have become available in combating infections, correcting metabolic defects, and in recognizing the tangible promise of forthcoming medical-related technology. The thrust of these innovations, and in particular pharmacological medications, has won out over age-old traditional ignorance and offered prospects of bringing numerous disease under therapeutic control. There has been accelerated development in medical research, as a consequence of which medicine itself has come to rest upon an expanding groundwork of scientific sophistication that provides a firm basis for improvement in patient care.

Not least in recent advances is the pioneer work of that small band of innovative physicians and colleagues who have contributed to the establishment of health communications and to the advance of medical information systems. It takes a great deal of patience, courage, and dedication, to work for years on the cutting edge of new ideas, especially in an historical environment in which, generally speaking, established physicians have been *non-believers*.

Within this framework of change, the contributors represented in this book have, often from their own resources, and almost always without the assistance of governmental agencies or corporate funds, expanded the desiderata for the basis and principles upon which contemporary, advanced, cost-effective and reliable computers for physicians are marketed.

An editor, generally speaking, must assume the responsibility or otherwise of the mission his book undertakes. In the domain of computer development this is no light task, for the field advances apace under different forces and in different paradigms recognising the economic conditions under which nationally different physicians practice or serve. It is difficult to compare systems or even to propose, on an *international* basis, an overall perfect model. Computers for physicians will relate to national philosophies, national psychologies, national priorities, and regional and national patient/physician relationships. To some

v

thinkers, irrespective of national background, the physician/patient relationship is a sacred cow, not to be desecrated by insensitive technology. The tradition and ethics of medicine is in some minds so deeply embedded in the past, and so well grounded in classical concepts of physician protection of patient privacy, confidentiality, and the purple and Godhead of the physician role, that information systems, flexible or not, appear to be repugnant and merit no claim in the practice of medicine.

To others, who might be quite prepared to evaluate potential systems in practice, the cost of the system is important. Litigation consequent upon machine systems may be feared, and medical recording in private practice is a source of other problems and unresolved issues relevant to the quality of medical care delivered.

Billing, patient registration, patient scheduling, accounting, and statistical reports have had variable appeal over the last 10 years. Special research committees in several nations have at various times been established to enquire into the economic advantages of various systems, e.g., PROMIS (Problem Oriented Medical Information System); COSTAR (Computer Stored Ambulatory Record); Kaiser-Permanente System in Oakland, California; CHAMPS at Canyon General Hospital in Anaheim, and so forth.

On national and international thresholds, transfer of patient data to central information banks has been of concern to the practicing physician, and national legislation such as that in Sweden, Canada, and the United States relevant to information derived from professional sources has added to the *non-believer* role.

Those who *do* believe may not be free of constraint. The system introduced for patient and office should not exceed the overhead cost physicians are normally called upon to pay for manual procedures. Systems based on inexpensive microcomputers do not have enough storage capacity. If the capacity is increased, the computer price no longer becomes acceptable. Time sharing features may not work with minicomputers in practice, and large time sharing systems may be beyond the comprehension and also the financial means of the majority of practitioners.

Yet curiously, experience confirms that most physicians, including *non-believers,* strongly agree that current manual systems used in doctor's offices are obsolete and cumbersome, and many believe that they are unduly costly, although the true cost is often hidden.

This state of affairs is rapidly improving. Research experiences, and the international range and variable economics from which the present authorship is drawn, obviously enough portrays variable viewpoints. The experience of a physician in Australia reasonably is different from that of a physician in Arkansas, in the United States.

Complexities and benefits each author relates will be relevant to his own national background, to regional policies, and to the practice of medicine to which he relates. In the United States, for example, in the 24 months between editorial submission and publication, remarkable advances have occurred, and major corporations have introduced much simplified systems — removing complexities, improving cost effectiveness, and considerably reducing implementation time. Recent advances, remarked by James Goddard,* now offer access to large-scale systems and data bases using a modem. This is becoming an important field and will be the area, in Goddard's view, with the greatest growth over the next few years. "It will open up an entirely new spectrum of information services to the physician's office: summaries of articles in the physician's areas of special interest which have been accessed by the National Library of Medicine during the previous week; information on new pharmaceuticals; drug interactions; adverse reaction information; post-graduate medical education programs, etc.

Today computers, (even low cost), are seldom awkward and are not all unreliable devices with circumscribed utility. In order to provide a brief overview for those health providers interested in computer use chapters in this book have been sequenced. The introductory material has been arranged to expose the physician to an understanding of how we have arrived at our current level of development. Subsequently the book presents principles to be followed, selection criteria, what the physician can look forward to with advanced systems, the ethical and legal issues as they are currently viewed, the state of the art in hospitals, and anecdotal experiences of computers seen through the developmental work of pioneering physicians.

The authors represented here have an international background, and generally speaking have cooperated with each other, in special relationships, correspondence, and common goals, over several years.

Some of the contributions presented here should be emphasized. Professor Gabrieli's chapter on the use of computers in medical practice should silence many critics of this field, since it moves away from the mechanistic routine functions of billing, scheduling, etc., and emphasizes applications related to diagnosis and therapy. Widespread application of his approach will have great impact on physician education and on the quality of care provided.

The chapter by Professor Annas on the ethics and legal aspects of computers in medicine will reassure physicians, many of whom, as just pointed out, have been concerned about these issues. Dr. Brandejs has, in a very concise fashion, set forth the design principles to be followed in an office system. His words should be heeded by any individual or group considering the lease or purchase of a system. Few physicians know enough about computers to appreciate the nuances and criteria for selection and use. The work of Dr. Brandejs, and many

---

*James Goddard, Personal Communication, July 1981.

of the other authors with whom he has personally worked, add clarity, and will, hopefully, introduce the full prospect of this very important field developed to enhance patient care by the practicing physician.

Stacey B. Day MD., PhD., DSc.
Clinical Professor of Medicine, Division of
Behavioral Medicine, Department of
Medicine, New York Medical College
Valhalla, New York

CONTENTS

Preface   v

1 Introduction to Computer-Oriented Health Informatics,
     by Stacey B. Day   1

2 Design Principles of Computer-Aided Physician's Office Systems,
     by Jan F. Brandejs   65

3 Criteria for Selection of a Feasible Medical System,
     by Peter V. Weston   75

4 "Praktice" – An Advanced Clinical Information System,
     by E. R. Gabrieli   88

5 Medical Privacy and Confidentiality,
     by George J. Annas   102

6 Computers in Hospitals,
     by Donald Fenna   125

7 The Computer in General Medical Practice,
     by Graeme R. Simpson   141

8 Experience With the Alpha Micro (AM 100) in a Doctor's Office,
     by Peter E. Levers   151

9 Improving Clinical Performance in General Practice with a $1500
Micro–System,
     by Robert A. Johnson   157

10 Doctor's Office Computers in the German Health System,
     by Erhard Geiss   172

Index   193

Computers For Medical Office And Patient Management

1
INTRODUCTION TO COMPUTER—ORIENTED HEALTH INFORMATICS

Stacey B. Day, New York

EVOLUTION OF SYSTEMS STRUCTURE THROUGH NUMBERS, INFORMATION USAGE, AND COMPUTER METHODOLOGIES

1. From Prehistory to the Concept of Zero

The story is told of the remarkable encyclopedist Diderot that, while at the Russian court, he was informed that a mathematician had established proof of the existence of God, and that it would be fitting if he would debate this issue with the philosopher. The tsaritsa had in fact commissioned the mathematician Euler to debate in public with Diderot. Before the assembled court, Euler gravely proclaimed

$$\frac{a + b^N}{N} = X$$

"from which God must exist" (Donc, Dieu existe, repondez). Regrettably, Diderot was quite unfamiliar with algebra. He experienced stage fright when confronted by a proposition in number and size language, became an object of ridicule (though he *was* an outstanding communicator), and left the royal patronage somewhat humiliated.

The point of the matter is that had he thought to suggest to Euler that they both communicate in the same language, or had he asked Euler to translate

$$\frac{a + b^N}{N} = X$$

and God, he would have asked, "How are the two sides of the equation related?"

Diderot, as a renowned encyclopedist and "information gatherer" was at fault. He showed himself to be limited of understanding in how to use knowledge content (in this case, the equation); and, most important, he revealed that he did not know the "language of mathematics." It would have been desirable for him, as a man of learning, to have enquired about this new language. What was it? How was it constructed? If it could be used to prove that God existed, it was clearly a remarkable language. All men must share this new knowledge. He, Diderot, the renowned encyclopedist, would consider it a sacred trust to pass on this extraordinary quantitative (size measurement) tongue that could describe an omnipotent qualitative image, the Deity! Instead, he made a fool of himself.

Lancelot Hogben many years ago stated the case in terms of much-needed appreciation, *science literacy,* so necessary for us all in an age of computers: "the plain man can understand scientific discoveries if they do not involve complicated measurements . . . . the plain man has not been taught to read and write *size language.* Three centuries ago, when priests conducted their services in Latin, protestant reformers founded grammar schools so that people could read the bible. The time has now come for another Reformation. People must learn to read and write the language of measurement so that they can understand the open bible of modern science" (Lancelot Hogben, 1936).

Of course, there was much lament. Today we still have senior administrators very much like the good Diderot. To the degree that they resort to the dictionary to find the revelation in such words as "algorithm," they shuffle in the tail wind of Edmund Burke, who conceived sorrowfully that Europe (and presumably the United States too), would become a "continent of calculators." Alas! It is *fait accompli.* The glory of man the calculating animal is a fact of modern life. He is here in his cultural flowering in a "welter of figures, cooking recipes, railway time tables, unemployment aggregates, fines, taxes, war debts, overtime schedules, speed limits, bowling averages" and a miscellany of "size measurements" described by Hogben over 40 years ago! Fortunately, except to the overestablished establishment, he is not a prisoner in his cultural and social inheritance, but has learned to speak and think in the language of numbers, as well as in the language of words.

That man does have need to codify and perfect rule of order (discipline) in his thinking, usefully determined partly by a system of hierarchical values, has certainly been known since the great *Code of Hammurabi* (of Babylon), 1800 B.C. This codex was applied to broad multidisciplinary realms including social classes (division of subjects of the realm into three designations, with freemen being the highest class), property, family solidarity, trial by ordeal, and criminal law established on the principle of *lex talionis* or law of retaliation (an eye for an eye).

With the guarantee of law there was stabilization of the realm. Other codes became possible. Nomadic tribal passages were phased out in favor of structure-oriented integrated societies based on agriculture, husbandry, commerce, and business, which interests invited and required "numbers and counting." The calculator became important in the affairs of mankind.

In fact civilized man had developed rudimentary symbols for numbers, and primitive numbering was possible via notches on wood, marks on pebbles, shells and stones, and use of tally sticks. The earliest device or instrument for counting was the abacus or "counting frame" possessed by the Chinese several centuries before Christ (1000 B.C.).

This fixed frame with beads remained the only instrument for counting for centuries. Though valuable it was relatively limited, since no conceptual vocabulary of numbers existed in antiquity. This vocabulary became possible when the ancient Hindus conceptualized the zero (0), about 100 B.C.

Hogben writes that "in the whole history of mathematics there has been no more revolutionary step than the one which the Hindus made when they invented the sign 0 to stand for the empty column of the counting frame." What essentially became possible was a vocabulary permitting mankind to add up on paper as well as on an abacus. This vocabulary developed hand in hand with social, cultural, number usage, and information needs as society grew.

The Hindu word for 0 is *sunya,* which means empty. Philosophical concepts of sunya and the *infinite* world had long prevailed in Indian thinking, and the infinity concept had been symbolized as two snakes (serpents of wisdom) embracing or devouring each other in an infinite whole or ∞ (two circles juxtaposed).

The epochal character of the nature of zero is well described by Laplace, one of the most exceptional of all mathematicians who have contributed to scientific knowledge, and the one who told Napoleon "that God is not a necessary hypothesis in natural science":

It is India that gave us the ingenious method of expressing numbers by means of ten symbols, each symbol receiving a value of position, as well as an absolute value; a profound and important idea which appears so simple to us now that we ignore its true merit, but its very simplicity, the great ease which it has lent to all computations, puts our arithmetic in the first rank of useful inventions.

Dantzig remarked, "Is it not equally strange that algebra, that cornerstone of modern mathematics, also originated in India . . . . ?"

Without the sunya or 0 concept, modern space vehicles would not exist, men would not have landed on the moon, and wise administrators behind the times would not be looking up the meaning of "algorithm" in a Computer Age!

Mathematically then 0 is a cipher. Then zero has the following properties:

$$a + 0 = a$$

$$a \times 0 = 0$$

Then if a is any number except 0:

$$a^\circ = 1$$

and

$$0/a = 0$$

Division by zero is undefined. Zero cannot be a divisor. Arabic scholars took the zero into the Levant and Byzantium under the transliteration zephyrum. It was carried by mercantile expansion to Italy where it took on such forms as zuero, zepiro, and zero. Borrowed by the French as zero, it was beneficently bestowed by them upon the Anglo-Saxon world as zero!

This, in an intellectual sense, completed the first phase of the evolution of systems structure, which can be chronologically represented as in Table 1. It is of interest to note that nearly all of the civilizations of antiquity contributed to the language of numbers and information usage, which advance was arrested by the onset of the Dark Ages. Between the birth of Christ and A.D. 1494, we have no record of any significant advance in enumeration methodology.

Table 1. Evolution of numbers, I.

Prehistory	
2000 B. C.	Codex of Hammurabi, King of Babylonia
1000 B. C.	Abacus frame (China)
	Babylonian clay tablets
	Egyptian Papyros
100 B. C.	Ancient Hindus conceptualized
	The Zero Concept
	Vocabulary of numbers begins
	Algebra as cornerstone of mathematics
After Christ	Arabic numbers
	Roman books (transcribed)

2. From the Concept of Zero to Numbers in Navigation and the Foundations of Modern Statistical Theory

The cultural exchanges of the early civilizations of course required systems of communication. At the primary level of exchange were the economic systems of barter and the migratory caravanserai, the early caravan passages between Europe, the Middle East, and the Indus Valley civilizations. With increasing commercial undertakings and the aggregations of regions into political states, power became a major primitive in the organization and development of societies. Enhancement of this power was sought, and increased by the opening up of sea routes and mercantile shipping lanes, particularly in the Mediterranean Sea and its associated civilizations. Trade routes brought migration, intermarriage, and transcultural communications. It is not surprising therefore that use of the Indian system of numerals passed via Arabic-speaking intermediates to the threshold of Western European knowledge. In fact adoption of this system of enumeration was perhaps the single most important imperative in the rise of science in Europe, and the determining factor in growth of science and technology in the sixteenth and seventeenth centuries. In a sense the medieval trade routes not only ensured that the potential for technology in the West would be facilitated; but by the process of expansion of these principles in mathematics, and by the rapid rise of marine fleets of West European nations themselves, the advent of future technology (and one might also say technocracies) was predictable centuries ago.

The foundation, then, of Indian algebra transmitted via Arabic schoolmasters to Western minds, culminating notably in the contributions of John Napier, led in 1614 to publication of collectivization or the mathematical invention of logarithms, a method of facilitating computation (*Mirifici Logarithmorum canonis descriptio,* 1614, and *Mirifici Logarithmorum canonis constructio,* 1619). This powerful thesis established a correspondence between an arithmetical and a geometrical progression. Let us arrive at this understanding by comparing simple algorithms for multiplying two numbers and adding the same two numbers. For example, 324 X 245 can be represented as:

$$
\begin{array}{r}
324 \\
\times\, 245 \\
\hline
648 \\
1296 \\
\underline{1620} \\
79{,}380
\end{array}
$$

If we add 324 to 245; we can express this as:

$$
\begin{array}{r}
324 \\
+245 \\
\hline
569
\end{array}
$$

Clearly the number of operations involved in multiplication is always greater than the number of operations involved in addition. In this example when we compare simple algorithms, for addition we have one operation, whereas for multiplication we have four operations.

It is quite obvious therefore that if we used very large numbers, the amount of labor, time, and effort involved in the mathematical procedure would be considerably increased. The invention of logarithms achieved both circumvention of unnecessary labor and economy of effort, by reducing all multiplication to the addition of two numbers. Briggs, who first compiled the tables that are now used, stated the case thus:

Logarithmes are numbers invented for the more easie working of questions in arithmetike and geometrie . . . by them all troublesome multiplications and divisions are avoided and performed only by addition instead of multiplication and by subtraction instead of division. The curious and laborious extraction of roots are also performed with great ease . . . .

The possibility of adding numbers that can be looked up in tables was not the only mathematical concern of Napier. In 1617, he published his *Rabdologiae, seu numerationis per virgulas libri duo,* in which he described ingenious methods of performing the fundamental operations of multiplication and division with small rods, which commonly came to be known as Napier's bones.

Pragmatic refining of the logarithmic tables was contributed by Henry Briggs, first professor of geometry in Gresham College, London. He proposed the alteration of the scale of logarithms from the hyperbolic form of Napier to one in which unity is assumed as the logarithm of the ratio of ten to one. In 1624 he published his *Arithmetica Logarithmica,* a work containing the logarithms of 30,000 natural numbers to 14 places of figure besides the index. (In effect, following discussion and agreement with Napier, Briggs calculated the first logarithms to the base 10 of all numbers from 1 to 1,000 correct to 14 decimal places.)

Within the same half century or so, and with the same intellectual vigor, further extraordinary contributions to developing mathematics were made by Blaise Pascal in France and Gottfried von Leibnitz, who was born at Leipzig.

Pascal, with a brilliantly perceptive mind, added to many dimensions of human thought. Between 1642 and 1644 he conceived and constructed an arithmetical machine that was in fact the first adding machine. The quality of his thought, perpetuated on the walls of the Musée de L'Homme in Paris, is evident in the spiritual and philosophic contributions he made, along with his mathematical studies:

L'homme n'est qu'un roseau, le plus faible de la nature, mais c'est un roseau pensant. Il ne faut pas que l'univers entier s'arme pour l'ecraser. Une vapeur, une goutte d'eau, suffit pour le tuer. Mais quand l'univers l'ecraserait, l'homme serrait encore plus noble que ce qui le tue, parce qu'il sait qu'il meurt, et l'avantage que l'univers a sur lui, l'univers n'en sait rien.

Later in Europe, Leibnitz, one of the major systematic thinkers of modern times, both as metaphysician and logician, independently developed the differential and integral calculus, versions of which were similar to George Boole's algebra. Leibnitz's interest in abstract logical calculi was due in part to the fact that he saw them as sketches for a syntax of ideal language (the so called *lingua characteristica universalis*). This concept he had harbored over long years, for he was imbued with the vision of an ideal language that would serve as a universal encyclopedia, summarizing all experiential and known human knowledge. In his day this was a dream. With the advent of future generations of computer methodology this visionary concept holds every prospect of becoming a reality.

If one reviews the three quarters of a century between Napier's bones and Leibnitz's vision of a universal encyclopedia (see Table 2), it becomes clear that these advances were linked with the general social and cultural advances occurring in the Europe of those times. Pascal's *Traité du triangle arithmetique,* which was in fact a fragment of the *De Alea Geometriae,* laid the foundations of the *calculus of probabilities.* Conceptually his entire mathematical work contributed to the foundation of modern statistical theory. The intellectual thrust of the century turned about methodologies for systemization, calibration, and the simplification of numbers toward *applied use.* Such applications of logic and number theory we see in the adding machine, the logarithmic tables, and the construction of logarithmic sines and tangents for the hundredth part of every degree. The trigonometry of tangents and secants was to mature. Mathematics was to give improved tables of navigation. Briggs alone contributed much to this applied area: *A Table To Find the Height of the Pole, the Magnetical Declination Being Given* (1602), *Tables for the Improvement of Navigation (etc.)* (1610), and a *Treatise on the North-West Passage to the South Sea* (1622).

This was the century of improving navigation. Developing sea power brought wide commercial gains, and naval expansion ensured and in some ways overruled land or territorial expansion as it had been known within the fixed limits of European national boundaries. The sea lanes offered prospects of commerce and colonization. Mathematics and applied mathematics ensured reasonably safe prospects via a combination of technology and power as an imperative of rule. In the sixteenth century British seamanship and British ship construction proved a powerful investment. The intellectual growth and evolution of numbers, the development of algebraic and trigonometric functions, and the first technology of computation, in association with British naval expansion, heralded the age of Elizabethan acquisitions.

Table 2. Evolution of numbers, II

1494	Luca Pacioli: Double-entry bookkeeping
1614	J. Napier's bones
1624	Briggs' logarithms + slide rule
1642	Blaise Pascal: The first adding machine
1694	Gottfried von Leibnitz: Calculating machine

The continuing evolution of man's mathematical heritage — updated now in the concepts of new, growing, and continually improving sophisticated computer series and advanced technology and navigation philosophy — has transformed the Elizabethan oceans of 1600 to the space oceans of the 1980s. The simple seagoing navigational craft of earlier times have become, in our day, simple space and satellite navigational craft, so that British naval expansion of 1600 has become American space exploration of the twentieth century. It is hardly surprising that the ships and power of one era have evolved into the space ships and power of another era, not withstanding the fact that it has taken man collectively four hundred years to comprehend basic mathematics that were always, in all time, at his command. As with all knowledge, progress becomes simply a matter of seeing. The computer as such is as much a child of the mathematics of the past as it is of the number language of the present.

3. From Pattern Concept to Analytic Machine and Modern Computer

The century between 1765 and 1865 saw many changes in the British domestic woolen cloth manufacturing systems of Yorkshire and the North of England. Wool was often in variable supply, and growth in the textile industry became dependent upon mechanized instrumentation. Uncertainty in supplies of much needed raw material was offset by the importation of wool from the Levant, the West Indies, and South America, and of cotton from the East Indian acquisitions, made available to England by securing more certain sea power. In fact, the nation was, during those years, undergoing critical changes of far-reaching import. In England industrial organization changed to factory systems; handwork became machine work; steam power appeared early in the eighteenth century, and the textile markets adapted to new supply sources — Australia, New Zealand, and South America as well as imperial possessions and the U. S. colonies.

In the same years that saw great improvements in the science of navigation, new and innovative technological machines became widely used in cloth manufacturing (see Table 3).

Table 3. Technological improvements in the textile industry

1735	Kay's flying shuttle
1767	Hargreave and the spinning jenny
1769	Arkwright and the water frame
1776	Crompton's mule (which combined the advantages of the spinning jenny and the water frame)
1785	Cartwright's power loom
1825	Robert's mule
1847	The Northrop loom

Of particular importance among the technological improvements was the *Jacquard attachment,* an automatic selective shedding device that permitted weavers to produce intricately designed fabrics and pictures of considerable size. The Jacquard device was in fact the first known pattern-making technology to be devised in industrial application. Invented in 1801, Jacquard's machine, though "secret," was rapidly pressed into service, and in Coventry alone there were, for example, 600 Jacquard machines in use by 1832. *From the point of view of the evolution of computers the punched card can be considered to have originated as the card with holes used in the Jacquard loom to control the weaving of complicated patterns composed of different-color threads. The Jacquard loom gave birth to the punched card.* With this innovation "control equipment" was born in the sense of *machine steps* whose sequence could determine outcome. The analytic machine of Babbage was later to be actuated by punched cards, and the sequence to be determined was a function of the order in which the cards were fed into the equipment. *Data* could be entered into the machine by such cards. *Information* (as intermediate results) could be placed "in store," and later "retrieved."

In a sense, the principle of the "modern" computer was at hand. The Jacquard loom, much used for working worsted, was power-operated from about 1833, and by midcentury had effectively proved its economic advantages in the textile industry.

Charles Babbage, who might in a sense be called the originator of the modern automatic computer, was born in Devon, England, in 1791. He was by aptitude a mechanician, and by profession a mathematician. His contributions to knowledge were many. In English mathematics he replaced the Newtonian dot notation in the calculus by the Leibnitzian D notation. He contrived several mathematical "tables," and in 1823 constructed a small machine that would tabulate up to eight decimals a function whose second differences were constant. In 1823 he obtained government support for a projected *difference engine,* which never in fact was finished. A machine based on this idea of Babbage was made in 1855 by Scheutz, a Stockholm firm.

In 1834 Babbage invented the principle of the analytical engine (Figure 1), the automatic computer of the twentieth century. He was in every way an unusual man, considered to be "eccentric" by his neighbors, and generally unappreciated by government. Although instrumental in founding the Astronomical (1820) and Statistical (1834) societies, Babbage received very little real appreciation until long after his death. Curiously, like many of the most innovative mathematicians of those centuries, Babbage had a remarkable religious strength, fostered in several philosophical concepts that originated from a desire to show that "the power and knowledge of the great Creator of matter and mind are unlimited." There is no doubt, absolutely none whatever, that the sophisticated electronic computers of our times are but embodiments of principles that Babbage laid

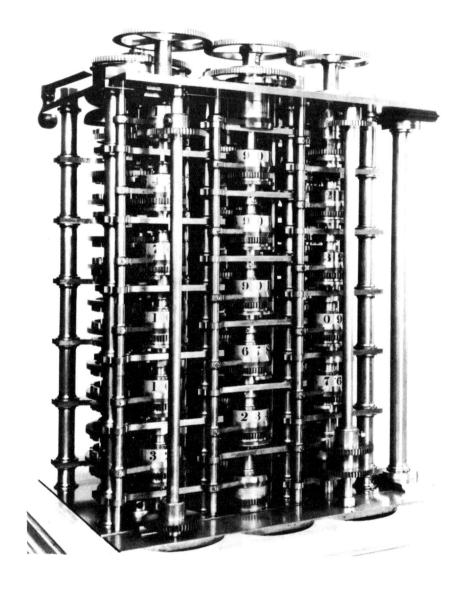

Figure 1. Babbage's analytical engine. (Reproduced with permission.)

down well over a century ago. Far ahead of his time, too far, Babbage's Difference Engine (as he called his "computer") gathered dust. In was unrecognized for the potential we accord it today.

In some ways the *feedback mechanism* with which Babbage's computer was equipped did not come of age until electronic tubes and circuits made feedback a feature of twentieth-century machines. Though much slower than electrons, the rods and gears of the feedback apparatus in Babbage's machine performed exactly the same function, which is considered by several cyberneticians of our times to be the very essence of intelligent operation (Jaki; A. M. Turing). Remarking on his Difference Engine No. 1, he said: "Calculating machines comprise various pieces of mechanism for assisting the human mind in executing the operation for arithmetic." His machine, Babbage said, admitted only "the direct processes of calculation." Lord Byron's daughter, Lady Lovelace, a gifted mathematician, remarked; "The Analytical Machine has no pretensions whatever to originate anything; it can do whatever we know how to order it to perform."

With this background and the idea of preprogramming machines through the use of punched cards (Jacquard, 1801), Dr. Herman Hollerith adopted the system to mechanize the U. S. Census of 1890, and in so doing accelerated the processing of collected data by punched-card use. As punched-card machines grew in popularity, Hollerith started the Tabulating Machine Company, which, following several mergers, became the International Business Machines Corporation (IBM) (see Table 4).

In cooperation with IBM, Professor H. Aiken, in 1944, 73 years after Babbage's death, developed the first digital computer. It was an electromechanical device with input and output on punched cards. The machine, named Harvard Mark I, did its calculations in decimal form, and found use principally in fields of scientific calculations. This machine was the first in a line leading to Mark IV, but the system was surpassed by a faster series of entirely electronic computers. The Electronic Numerical Integrator and Calculator (ENIAC), built in 1945, was a

Table 4. Evolution of numbers, III

1801	Joseph M. Jacquard: Use of punched strips (punch cards)
1812	Charles Babbage invented the difference engine
1830	Charles Babbage conceived and began the analytic machine
1854	George Boole described the Laws of Thought
1880	Dr. Herman Hollerith developed the unit punch card
1900	Hollerith sorting machine invented
1903	Hollerith Tabulating Machines Co.
1905	J. Powers
1911	Remington-Rand founded
1912	IBM founded

massive machine containing 18,000 vacuum tubes and weighing 30 tons. Capable of performing 300 multiplications per second, it was used initially for the solution of ballistics problems, mathematics related to atomic energy problems, and associated computations, until in 1956 it was retired to the Smithsonian Institute.

Edvac (Electronic Discrete Variable Automatic Computer), the first computer that did not require programs to be externally wired by hand, became operational in 1952 and was in service until 1962.

UNIVAC I, the first commercially available computer (Universal Automatic Calculator), was produced by Sperry Rand Corporation in 1951. This was the first general-purpose computer for data processing with the capability of storing and manipulating both digits and characters. Input and output used magnetic tape, and data were input through a keyboard or punched cards. This computer design was phased out in 1958. (See Table 5 for computer generations.)

The computer is a general-purpose tool capable of facilitating a variety of programs to problem-solve. Its usefulness lies in a wide range of capabilities, as conceived in principle over the last two centuries. Perhaps the most obvious merit of the concept, always recognized, is the speed at which the machine components (gears or electronics) can permit function. Although it is not yet independent of human direction, once given a problem and a set of instructions, the computer can solve that challenge without further human intervention. Once entered, a set of instructions is stored by the computer and can be utilized repeatedly for problem solving. It is interesting to realize that the computer can be put to constant use and is immune from fatigue. Unlike the human, it cannot enter into interpersonal communications or relationships, and at the present limits of our knowledge, it cannot verify for error. Such advantages as the computer possesses are exceptionally functions of its fast circuits. The human brain in comparison, while having a vast range of activity, is characterized by slow

Table 5. Computer generations

First generation: 1944–54	Relays, vacuum tubes, drums, switches Acoustic delays
Second generation: 1955–60	Electrostatic memory transistors Printed circuits
Third generation: 1961–70	Thin film memory Ferrit circuits Integrated ceramic base
Fourth generation: 1970–75	LSI Circuits Large-scale integrative
Fourth/fifth generation: 1970–80	Memory sheets (1980) Bubble memory

circuits. However, in some respects the brain is still superior to the computer. This is evident in pattern recognition, in which the brain is infinitely superior to most computers, which do not easily recognize patterns. Obviously optimum strategies require combining or augmenting human skills and computer technology via effective interfaces or "language" or communication "codes."

Although computer systems differ according to needs and application, certain generalizations are useful in defining specific portions of the system. *Input* is the communication information entered by the user to the computer. This information may be entered in the physical form of a punched card, via a terminal, or via a tape reader. *Output* is mediated by communication and transmission of information in the opposite direction, again usually via a terminal, line printer, or other print-out device. External to the computer is the *file* section, which may be in the form of a drum, disc, or magnetic tape. Within the computer is the *memory,* the control section, and the logic unit. The main memory holds the information for the control unit which derives the flow of data to the output and processing units.

Shipton has remarked that:

at the present time modern computers are beginning to look like biological systems . . . the architectural chart of modern machines is becoming essentially a network of devices interconnected and so designed that an enormous amount of "pre-processing" of data goes on at the periphery of the main computer. In other words, the modern computer is looking more and more like an interconnected network of smaller machines, each enjoying a substantial amount of autonomy. This use of pre-processing is a characteristic of sensory nervous systems . . . there remains the tantalizing problem of how biological memory is organized. We know that there are several levels; for example, that short term memories, i.e. memories of recent events, can be obliterated by illness or injury without much change in the recall of events knowledge obtained earlier. About all that can be said with certainty is that it does not depend on binary storage in "all or none" switching circuits. Even the vast numbers of such elements within the brain would be inadequate to account for the richness of human memory . . . the question of how the computer designer may benefit from evolutionary processes is of great interest.

Much of the value of the computer resides in the purpose of the data analysis it is able to perform. Data analysis constitutes a principal purpose of research itself, if by research we understand primary target goals to include obtaining data with the view to entering them into the total body of human knowledge; if we suppose that included in research goals is the prospect of discovery; and if we expect that research should include as a construct a need for validation of data —

which may be in various forms, hypotheses, results, confirmation of results, and so on.

Depending on the users' needs and the computer capability, a broad variety of functions is possible. These may include use of computers in such tasks as modelling systems (we might expect a model to organize complex data, simulate experiments we cannot possibly do — war games are a good example, and permit retrieval of parameters from data that may be more important than the data themselves are); explorations in Artificial Intelligence and applied epistemology (knowledge engineering, linguistic command comprehension, symbol data capture and analysis, and examination of knowledge-based systems); phenomenological supports (graphics may aid hypotheses?); and interactive graphics, which might include such tasks as statistical sampling, relating data bases to health care delivery, and in such areas of investigation as may deal with pharmacological interventions on neurocerebral pathways.

HANDLING INFORMATION

1. Human Information Processing

As we have seen, as society became more complex, new knowledge paved the way to more sophisticated and more readily available methods for manipulation and storage of information. In our present societies we have adapted the computer to problem-solve these needs. By and large, human information processing concerns three types of records: those related to administration; those related to intelligence — information — knowledge; and those related to statistical records. Since the computer is a nonmoral synthesis of responsive electronic components, it is unable to question the motives of its users. (Ethical aspects of privacy and confidentiality are discussed in Chapter 5.)

There have been tendencies to develop coordinated computer systems leading to concentration of data in central files or databanks. Such databanks invoke questions of data security and need of ways to limit access to such databanks.

There seems little doubt that increasingly complex records, and in infinitely culturally integrated earth with pluricausal needs and complex societal structures, will come to depend more and more upon computer technologies. This interaction will require society vs. technology trade-offs: Society on the one hand will perforce have to yield some personal rights of information in order to receive broader benefits from accumulated data representing whole communities. Inherent in such "whole data" is potential information/knowledge for improved health.

2. Information Retrieval

From a classical viewpoint, information systems may be structured at two levels: information storage and retrieval systems (ISR) and control management information systems (MIS). Descriptions of these systems are well covered in published materials. Leach cites over 5000 items available on surveys of bibliography on information storage alone. Despite this extraordinary surfeit of literature, she states that "the major goal of any information system, a satisfied user, has almost been omitted from the research, analysis, design and implementation processes." Bishoff, in his work "Die Information Lawine," emphasizing need for effective information storage and retrieval systems, points out that in the following areas a doubling of knowledge accumulates in the times given:

General information	Every 10 years
Chemical information	Every 8 years
Information in electronics	Every 5 years
Information on space	Every 3 years

King points out that it took *Chemical Abstracts* 30 years to publish its first million abstracts; 18 years to publish its second million; 8 years to publish its third million; 4 years to publish its fourth million, and less than 3 years to publish its fifth million. Still the exponential growth of chemical (and, in general, scientific research) literature continues. Price has pointed out, moreover, that the growth rate of scientific journals has been an exponential function of time for the past 200 years. This state of affairs has led to efforts to design improved strategies of cooperation between primary and secondary publishers in order to eliminate duplication.

Strategies for handling, analyzing, and publishing biological data must take into account difficulties in locating data, time expended in searching indexes, conflicting values of choice in subjects, and variable viewpoints on ways of assembling, evaluating, and disseminating data. The publications of Altman, Challinor, Marcy, and King usefully review features of these problems.

3. Continuous Modelling Systems

North American Society is approaching that stage in which human service delivery systems will prevail over industrial production (Brandejs, 1978a). This type of society has come to be known as the postindustrial society. With the emergence of computers during World War II, many new scientific techniques were evolved to test real or imaginary situations in order to develop operational concepts and optional directions for the postwar industrial technocracy. This type of represen- tation is called *modelling*. Operations research, commonly called OR, is possibly the most widespread application science for models research, undertaking quanti- tative studies of operations in action. Work in operations research has been pro- ductive of such theoretical models of human activity as encountered in queuing theory, and in systems and bioengineering problems in hospitals, factories, and governments.

In general, models of systems are subjective, based on individual assumptions, and are concerned with results. Because human variability strongly influences the outcome of any single operation within a modelled system, the theory of probability provides the basis of many of the mathematical models. A wide variety of statistical application techniques − including cluster analysis, least mean square methods, factor analysis, discriminant analysis, and decision − theoretic approaches, as well as probabilistic models and nonprobabilistic symptom − vector- based methods for diagnosis − have been used in such areas as, for example, mathematical modelling techniques for diagnosis of disease. Over the last 15 years in particular, various applications of the Bayes therorem with its strong assumption for statistical independence of disease-associated symptoms have predominated in problem-solving approaches to clinical decision processing. This application of the Bayes theorem in medical diagnosis is largely due to the work of Ledley and Lusted.

In general, problem situations and, more specifically, decision problems can be represented and analyzed in terms of graphs and trees. The decision point may be either a decision state (action tree) or a decision problem (goal tree). In the problem-solving literature the goal tree structure corresponds to the problem- reduction representation, while the action tree corresponds to the state-space representation.

It is important to remember that problem-solving knowledge and algorithms facilitate each other. Human experts are of great importance and highly valued because they have the potential to be good problem solvers. Slamecka has appropriately remarked that "human problem solving expertise today is at an all-time premium in all professions but particularly in health care." This human knowledge is reinforced by those data recorded and stored in extensive physical documentation banks. One of the emerging powerful new directions in health care is the design and development of computer-based "expert systems" (Gorry, 1974), capable of deploying elements of the problem-solving expertise normally associated with humans.

4. Machine Intelligence

Initial interest in the field of artificial intelligence commenced with the computer science studies of A. M. Turing, who, in 1950, suggested that a machine is intelligent if an individual is unable to decide whether he is interacting with a computer or with another human using a teletype.

Langer and Brandejs suggest that a broad definition of artificial intelligence (AI) might be proposed in the limits of "the intelligence of any machine that performs a task that a century ago would have been considered a uniquely human intellectual ability." Pragmatically the machine is usually a digital computer or is controlled by a digital computer, and requires that the task involve symbolic reasoning or "thinking" rather than arithmetic calculations or information storage and retrieval.

Such a definition should, I think, be augmented to take into account the question "What is a Machine?" To be sure, artificial intelligence embraces an area of computer science research. But it would be useful to emphasize that this research is focused on knowledge-based systems comprehending both general and symbolic knowledge of the world as one of its fundamental goals. In this sense AI is goal-oriented toward intelligent action guided by knowledge of the world. In a sense AI is *knowledge engineering,* and requires among many understandings interpretation of how symbols come to have meaning.

Jaki, in his text *Brian, Mind and Computer,* has remarked that "the ideal machine of cybernetics is a machine capable of imitating or reproducing those externally observed behaviors that can be described in a finite number of words." He bases this statement on a combination of Turing's definition of a machine and of the analysis of the model of the nervous system by McCulloch and Pitts. *But what is a machine?* Turing has defined what he called a "universal machine" in his article "On Computable Numbers With An Application to the Entscheidungs Problem," a good nontechnical paraphrase of which has been given by N. Morary as: "If we have a system which can be in one of several states, together with a list of those states, and the rules for getting from one state to another, then we have a machine." This, of course, raises the question of the difference that exists between behavior and experience observed in animals (including man) and in machines (which may be programmed). Can man enter into the artificial mind? Could any designer build a machine, that to use Jaki's words, "assisted by the editorial board of the *Oxford Book of English Verse* . . . (demonstrates) . . . an ability of poetic discrimination"? M. V. Wilkes, director of the Mathematical Laboratories at Cambridge University, has moved toward resolving this question by suggesting "a bright future for machines in executive capacities, but I do not see them behaving like human beings."

The critical point is, I think, that in the present state of our interpretation of knowledge, machines *can* discriminate between quantities, but are presently not themselves each uniquely able to perceive those intellectual sensations and expressions that we commonly recognize to be manifest in poetry, the fine arts, and the emotional passions of men. The truth is that the computer is the finest of uniquely *quantitative* discriminators, but does not have "personal" qualitative discriminatory talents which functionally set men apart from all other known life forms.

The application areas that presently encompass artificial intelligence include: game playing; mathematical, scientific, and engineering aids; automatic theorem proving; automatic programming; robots; machine vision; natural language systems; and information-processing psychology. In effect, artificial intelligence bears on problems of describing information so that it can be used by a computer to perform tasks that require intelligence in humans. This knowledge might be referred to as *common sense knowledge,* heuristic knowledge, or informal knowledge of the world rather than logic or mathematical knowledge.

From the point of view of symbolic problem solving, we might consider interpreting speech which we could conceive as complex signal data. Speech-understanding research, appreciating issues of AI, might include such mechanisms as puzzles, chess games, speech, vision, and concepts of molecular structure, in some areas of which matrix data oblige computers to be superfast, as required say by response rates in speech and vision. Generally speaking, any system that has to recognize a large amount of data coming in needs high-speed signal-processing capabilities which may take such forms as graphical output or hard-copy output. A chess master, for example, may have a *pattern* vocabulary of 50,000 abstract patterns, and performance is related to task and knowledge. Hearsay systems as in speech and computer science research may involve divers sources of knowledge: *acoustic, lexicon, syntax, vocabulary, pragmatics,* and *semantics,* for example. Again syntax or syntactic theory may involve use of other sources of knowledge. The lexicon might involve phonetics, acousticophonetic knowledge, and probabilistic research, as well as entries into the lexicon; the recognition process would involve syntax, semantics, acoustic phonetics, and so forth. Knowledge sources are utilized to work with each other. In this sense knowledge-based systems must establish interrelated ways of working together, the cooperative and integrated result of their efforts, so to speak, making possible the solution of a single task.

The expression of information will depend in part on how the knowledge is used. Consider the amount of information in a video picture. How much information can the brain take up? How much, in terms of "bits of information" from the picture, may friend to friend, so to say, be taken up as data per second? Put otherwise, when you look at a picture, how much or how many "bits of information" does any given individual take in? What are the processes involved? How do we apportion combination, synergy, graphics display?

These directions of research in human and machine information processing usefully exemplify the ways and extent to which algorithmic machines and programs can best be used to aid the heuristic abilities of the human mind. Problem solving by machine thus requires insight in how to use knowledge, and necessitates strategies of using small amounts of knowledge to overcome constraints in the environment. In fact, heuristic research at its best involves augmentation or change of form of knowledge. We become concerned with ways and methodologies by which knowledge is transformed, or by which different kinds of knowledge collaborate and synthesize. Knowledge management and *relevance* and appropriateness of any single piece of knowledge are all of concern in determining outcomes and reactions.

One might apply this concept to modern medicine on the grounds that the discipline has become so complex that no single individual can incorporate all medical knowledge into his decision-making powers. Thus such a system as MYCIN, for example, which incorporates diagnostic, prognostic, therapeutic, and educational planning, has been investigated with a view to serving as a wise decision-making selector for a patient with a bacterial infection, on the grounds that physicians often do not choose antimicrobial therapy wisely, and often prescribe in a less than satisfactory clinical way.

The study of human problem-solving processes in the domain of medicine and health must be considered as an important research area in health informatics.

5. Cybernetics

The development of the principles of the computer inevitably brought to the fore questions of *control systems* or information management systems with capability to manipulate information. Control systems are required to manipulate and control events in the real world. *Input* into the system therefore must represent information about events that are taking place and situations that exist in the real world. *Output* is not information for human use, but rather *decisions* to be implemented by humans or by other machines in order to modify or institute new events. *The broad general area for the theoretical basis of automatic control has been called cybernetics.*

The word "cybernetics" was introduced into the vocabulary of science of control and communication processes in both animals and machines by Norbert Weiner, a highly original American-born mathematician with extraordinary insight into abstract mathematics, in 1948. This word Weiner derived from the Greek *kybernetes,* which means "steersman." It is quite different from "la cybernetique" of Ampere, which in military reference we today call logistics, "the science of general staff planning, or, more generally, the science of rational government administration."

Information Input. Unger has reasonably pointed out the extraordinarily varied roots of cybernetic activity, which is unquestionably wide and interdisciplinary in content. It is an activity in which, to cite Unger, "anatomists, physiologists, communications engineers, control engineers, and last but not least mathematicians, work together." The field of cybernetics deals with the theory of such systems as the nerve networks in animals, electronic computing machines, servo systems for the automatic control of machinery, and other information-processing systems. In this sense cybernetics seeks to find features common to these diverse disciplines. The dominant feature in cybernetics is that information is treated as a statistical quality. It might be remarked that wisely conducted science ensures types of study that statistically provide the maximum possible amount of information from the data obtained in experimental research. The implication is clear. In extracting the total information, means must be at hand to measure its content. Information must be reckoned in "degrees of freedom of the variability of the result" (Unger). The scientist must orient his thinking to understand that information can and must be measured. This is a relatively new psychophysiologic mind construct that has been developed markedly in post-World War II society.*

This idea of measuring information owes much to the pioneer work of Claude Shannon at Bell Telephone Laboratories. He was one of the first to succeed in finding a theoretical measure of information.

From the viewpoint of pure mathematics, it was principally the Russian researchers Chintchin, Kolmogoroff, Jaglom, and Jaglom who consolidated measurement of information. The importance of this process of mathematization cannot be overemphasized. These contributions and this approach indicate an important area for development in medicine and biology. Mathematization of the sciences post World War II made certain that biology is now firmly directed toward becoming a *quantitative* science (rather than, as in the past, relying solely on qualitative constructs) and has made possible new philosophical vistas for the development of theoretical biology.

This section will consider briefly only a few areas of cybernetics as applied to medicine and the problem of machine diagnosis.

Special contributions to this field have been made by Vishnevskiy, Artobolevskiy, and Bykovskiy in the Soviet Union and by Gorry and Otto Barnett in the United States.

Soviet scientists particularly have given attention to the use of methods in the theory of automatic control in medicine and biology. Vishnevskiy has perceptively pointed out

that the word "automation" does not mean the exclusion of man from the sphere of this activity and his replacement by a machine, but the planning of new and more precise methods of diagnosis which are based on the use of electronic mathematical machines operated by man and which are his equip-

---

*Although certainly and clearly recognized and emphasized over 50 years ago by Sir Wilfred Trotter in Great Britain.

ment for expanding the potentials in this field. The use of computers in diagnosis is important in those cases when it is a component of the general control scheme. This holds, for example, in medicine, where we are confronted with the problem of analyzing a vast amount of medical information and evaluating a constantly changing situation on the basis of this analysis selecting the optimal therapy plans, etc.

Vishnevskiy et al. have published a monograph devoted to investigations of one of the central problems in medical cybernetics − the problem of machine diagnosis. This text is worth consulting by those who address themselves to this area of medical communications. Herbert Sherman, of the Lincoln Laboratories, M.I.T., has remarked that the body of data stored at the Vishnevskiy Institute may well serve as a reference set against which all subsequent data bases for Bayesian diagnosis may be compared. As a theoretical foundation for diagnostic choice, Bayesian probability proposes that in a condition of decision under risk, understanding the rate of change of state of the disease may be open to the decision process. In an attempt to obtain probability occurrence from direct or indirect parameters, if a priori probabilities are available, and data can be gathered that will permit the conversion of a priori probabilities to a posteriori probabilities, then the solution obtained by evaluating the alternatives using the a posteriori probabilities is identical to the Bayes strategy.

It is almost inevitable that such far-reaching advances in mathematics and technology will bring in their wake fundamental and no less critical problems of social conscience and ethics. Norbert Weiner himself was much aware of the potential of his newborn "child." He was frequently challenged by such questions as whether his "thinking robots" constituted a threat to man. In 1960 Weiner himself took pains to note that "the human brain is a far more efficient control apparatus when we come to higher areas of logic." In *God and Golem* he warned against imagining the future as a state where mechanical slaves would allow men to rest from thinking. In his writing *The Human Use of Human Beings*, Weiner was sensitive to so-called human decisions entrusted to "Tin Mikes" (his name for the machines). Sociologists like Andreski have argued that despite Weiner's *Human Use of Human Beings* (control and communications in the animal and the machine), and "despite its undeniable potentialities, up till now the chief use of cybernetic terms in the study of politics and society has been to blind the reader with pseudo-science and to give spurious weight to ponderous platitudes."

Analogies between society and machines will continue into the future. Cybernetic viewpoints in sociology will be further debated. Such discussions as befit cybernetics, computers, and the thought and social process should be aided by reference to sources in the literature (Weiner, Jaki, Andreski, etc.).

It may be remarked that social Darwinism, or, as I have preferred to term it, biosocial development, will increasingly warrant our serious concern; for society is a system in which processes of adaptation and diversity, as well as of equilibrium, in both individuals and the community as a whole, must encompass acceptance of continuing ideas of control and of interaction with regulating systems. These ideas are embodied in biopsychosocial health and growth.

6. Hardware

Hardware features in a general sense include analog computers, digital computers, input/output devices, and microprocessors. The computer system consists of both electronic elements and mechanical parts. The central processing unit consists almost entirely of electronic elements such as transistors, resistors, and diodes, whereas most input/output equipment and file storage devices contain both electronic components and parts that move mechanically. The electronic circuits of the computer are designed to control the timing, strength, and frequency of electrical impulses that operate the computer system. A computer is thus seen to be an electronic computational device having internal storage, a stored program of instructions, and the capacity for modification of the instructions in response to a command to execute the program. There are two main types of computer, *digital* and *analog.* The digital computer operates essentially by counting. All quantities are expressed as numbers. The analog computer operates by measuring voltages which are read from meters. Computers that combine features of both analog and digital types are called *hybrid* computers. In the general way in which we speak of "computers," almost all present-day machines are electronic and are in fact digital computers.

Table 6 reviews computer systems in use during 1944-73. (See also Figure 2.)

7. Programming Languages

Language is the communications code by which any given problem is presented to the computer for solution. Available languages range from low-level machine language written in binary codes to sophisticated and elegant languages whose single statements incorporate the functions of many lower-level language statements.

Since all languages are broken down into basic machine language, it is useful to review the common binary language of simple machines. In these machines instructions and numbers are represented as strings of binary digits or "bits." The first programs were written entirely in this form until it was realized how cumbersome the technique was. Gradually programmers developed higher language levels so that by 1957 A-2, A-3, PRINT, and BACAIC had appeared.

These languages proved to have rigid formats, and were gradually replaced between 1960 and 1965 by machine-independent languages. Present-day successful and widely used languages include FORTRAN, BASIC, PL/1, and COBOL; but

Table 6. Computer systems, 1944–73

1944-45	1951	1955	1959	1961-69	1972-73
MARK I	ENIAC	UNIVAC SS 80	IBM 1440	CDC 6600	SUPER-
MARK II	EDVAC	IBM 1401	IBM 1460	GE 415/425	COMPUTERS
ZUSE 23	UNIVAC I	RCA 501	GE 215	HONEYWELL 200	BURROUGHS 850
MARK III	IBM 650	CDC 1604	UNIVAC 1050	IBM 360/40	SCDC 6700
	IBM 702	NCR 390	IBM 7094 11	IBM 360/50	IBM 360/92
		UNIVAC III	RCA 3301	RCA SPECTRA 70	ICL 1908 A
		CDC 160		UNIVAC 1108(11)	
		IBM 7040		IBM 360/67	
		HONEYWELL 1800			
		CDC 3600			
		IBM 7010			

SPEED	SPEED	SPEED	SPEED	SPEED
200 revol min.	10^{-3} $\frac{1}{1,000,000}$	10^{-6}	$\frac{1}{1,000,000,000}$	1,000,000,000,000
$\frac{1}{1,000}$ MILLISECOND 10^{-3}	MICROSECOND $= 10^{-6}$	$=$ SEC,	NANOSECOND $= 10^{-9}$	PICOSECOND $= 10^{-12}$

with continual advances being made in computer technology, continual improvements and updating are necessary not only for the programming languages, but also in programming theory and technology, and our understanding of the hardware itself.

It is useful to recognize that while computers provide the capability to make rapid calculations, search large files, compare and make decisions, and send messages via communication links to scattered terminals, the organization of

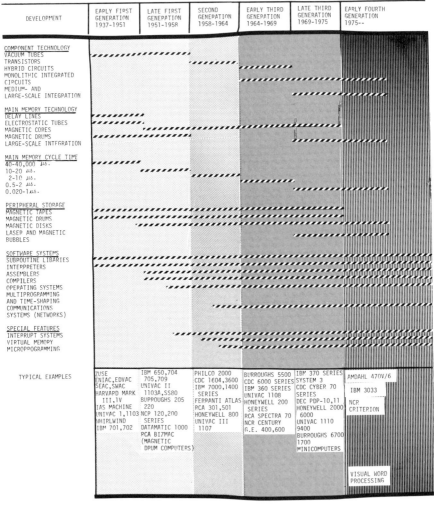

Figure 2. Computer generations.

these capabilities into a coherent system capable of problem solving depends on computer programs. Programs as such have been given the name *software* to indicate that they are distinct from but related to "hardware." Software includes not only the computer programs but also their documentation, and the training required for people to use the total system and to operate and maintain the programs. The following brief descriptions of specialized languages suggest that, at the present time, computer specialists have not succeeded in developing a *universal* language. Those concerned with practical needs should devote themselves to study of primary descriptions of the following specialized languages. This whole area is one of vast potential and provides extraordinary scope for the theoretical derivation of new, better, and more efficient methodologies in programming techniques and theory.

FORTRAN. One of the first of the major high-level languages to be developed was FORTRAN, IBM's Formula Translating system, first discussed in 1954. It was developed by 1957 for the IBM 704 computer and was intended for use in mathematical and numeric problems having provision for the handling of many variables and the computation of formulae. The original FORTRAN, a relatively machine-dependent language, was slowly developed into FORTRAN IV, which first appeared in 1962. It is natural in its algebraic notation, which is its major attraction as a computational language, and it is easy to learn.

FORTRAN's technical characteristics include a character set consisting of a full alphabet, the ten digits, and ten other symbols. Variable names consist of a letter followed by up to four alphanumeric characters and up to two subscripts with special provisions that make all variables beginning with the letters I, J, K, L, M, or N integers. It has a library of mathematical functions and provision for the calling of subroutines within programs. Because almost all aspects of FORTRAN have been duplicated and in many cases improved upon in recent years, its major importance lies in the fact that it is easy to learn and that it was the first language developed that was usable on the machines available at the time.

BASIC. BASIC (Beginners All-purpose Symbolic Instruction Code) is very similar to FORTRAN and is also a very simple language for the learner. It was developed at Dartmouth College in 1965 by John Kemeny and Thomas Kurtz as on online programming language intended specifically for students, but it has been found useful in various business and industrial applications. It is very similar in many ways to FORTRAN with one of the distinctions being that it allows only two-character variable names (a letter followed by a digit), has no integer variables, and, apart from supplying a library of functions, provides for user-defined functions. BASIC consists of two types of online commands: those that call for some function of the computer, such as RUN or LIST a program, and the program statements involving calculation or input/output functions within the program while the programmer is given extensive computing capabilities. Using a relatively small range of statements, the programmer is given extensive computing capabilities. The statements are of several types: arithmetic, logic, input and output, loop, and function and subroutines. All statements in BASIC programs are preceded by a statement number, and the program runs in ascending order of the numbers. Following each number is an English word defining the type of statement and then the numbers or variables involved in the statements. BASIC's main importance lies in its simplicity yet wide applicability, and the fact that it is an online system involving direct interaction between the user and the computer from a terminal keyboard. This allows the programmer much faster and easier editing and debugging capabilities than are available on any batch system, and thus increases its capabilities as a learning system.

PL/1. PL/1 (Programming Language 1) is the most modern of the languages discussed here. Many people found FORTRAN limited in some of its alphanumeric data-handling capabilities, and work was done within IBM to remedy this problem. At first, attempts were made toward the extension of the FORTRAN IV system itself, but this was found to be impractical. Thus, after a committee study of several other languages, including COBOL and ALGOL, the PL/1 language was produced in 1964.

A little later Allen-Babcock Computing Inc. developed RUSH, an online language based on PL/1, whose statements are, in fact, a subset of PL/1. PL/1 itself was found to be very successful, and it was thought by some that it would fulfill its original objective of replacing FORTRAN, COBOL, and the other major languages.

The technical characteristics of PL/1 include two character sets, one of 60 characters and another of 48 characters in which some of the symbols in the larger set are replaced by letters. Its complexity and wide range of uses arise from a very large variety of statements available to the programmer and a vast library of preprogrammed functions. It attempts to bring together all the desirable features of the major languages such as good data-handling capabilities, manipulation of matrices and arrays, and good computational facilities. As a result it offers the experienced programmer extremely powerful tools but is at the same time very complicated for the beginner. It is possible, however, to write programs using only a portion of the capabilities available. Another shortcoming of PL/1 is that while its programs tend to be relatively short in length, the complexity of the language itself requires a very large compiler for their processing. Nevertheless, PL/1 is growing in popularity and is probably the best of the attempts to provide the capabilities of many specialized languages within one language.

COBOL. Of the languages so far discussed, none approaches natural English as closely as does COBOL (Common Business Oriented Language). COBOL was created as the result of the work of a committee of representatives of a large group of users and manufacturers and first appeared in 1960. As indicated by its name, COBOL was developed for use in businesses and has good data-handling capabilities such as documentation and table creation. A COBOL program consists of four distinct sections: the identification division, the environment division, the data division, and the procedure division. The identification division merely holds the program name and comments. The environment division assigns the hardware that is used in execution. The procedure division defines the procedures that are to be performed on the files and data described in the data division of the program. COBOL is the first English-like language to be able to handle files and yet still remain relatively machine-independent. Moreover, its approximate likeness to English makes it relatively easy to learn and easy to read.

8. Network Synthesis

With our present knowledge, the application of network synthesis, and in particular queuing network theory, that appears most relevant to health problems is in a primitive and rudimentary state of research. While network design is considerably advanced and sophisticated in many areas of engineering, and simple techniques like the partial fraction method, the continued fraction method, and the Darlington synthesis commonly used in 1-port impedance synthesis are valuable approaches to mathematical and engineering problems, the vocabulary jargons and conceptual applications are difficult to translate for audiences of nonmathematicians, nonengineers, and nonphysicists.

Notwithstanding the difficulties posed by drawing mathematical boundaries, it is certain that the applicability of network to medical problems will be successfully advanced within the next decade. As interdisciplinary strategies improve and team work takes precedence over research chanteclairs and professorial stardom, interaction between medicine, science, mathematics, and engineering will permit the crystallization and opening up of important field questions.

A *network* may be regarded as a set of objects interconnecting with one another in a predetermined fashion. They are, usually, identifiable input and/or output quantities (e.g., in the case of an electrical network the objects are resistors, capacitors, inductors, gyrators, transformers), interconnecting according to certain prescribed fashions. The input and output are usually voltages and/or currents. *In the case of medical facilities, the objects may be doctors, X-ray departments, specialist consultants, etc.,* and the interconnections are taken to be routes that the patients pass through; *the input and output quantities are patients* (Mbaeyi, 1978).

There are two distinct disciplines within the study of networks:

1. *Network analysis:* One is interested in understanding the behavior of a given network and how it responds to stimuli or input.
2. *Network synthesis:* One is interested in finding a network that will furnish a given behavior when it is inserted in the path of a stimulus.

Classically linear electrical networks present a relatively fully developed and accessible theory of synthesis along this prescription. In linear electrical network studies, the input and output quantities are usually currents and voltages, and transfer characteristics, changes of amplitude of input and output signals, are easily defined. These principles form a reasonable basis for projections for future use in problems relevant to health care. They may find important and valuable use in assisting the Third World countries, who already have critical unbalanced distributions of essential social resources such as are related to health and health care, to transpose unfavorable conditions in attempts to catch up with the industrialized world.

Some simple illustrations of contemporary network design may serve to show the potential usefulness of these strategies. For example, Figure 3 illustrates the Chikatetsu Rosenzu or plan of the metropolitan underground railway, Tokyo. Nihonbashi Station in east-central Tokyo (circled) stands near the point from which all distances in Japan are calculated.

Transferring these principles one might consider developing a country with a network of public health services. All cities, towns, and villages would first be transformed into points. Such points, it is assumed, would be interconnected, as by roads, railway lines, transport systems, or other communications links. By mathematical techniques we can construct hypothetical *directed graphs,* for example (ones on which certain directions must be followed); and interlocking numbers of directed graphs possessing specific focal (or starting) points, we can derive networks that permit information to be transmitted across the network.

Such a basis allows assemblages as patterns of communication until a whole country is covered with a series of networks, which can be interrelated and controlled by a major nodal center. Presupposing that a country has the will to set up a health network, this oversimplified exposition can be formulated and optimized into mathematical functions, which when studied by intellectual play known as combinatorial games help establish the best and most useful possibilities available.

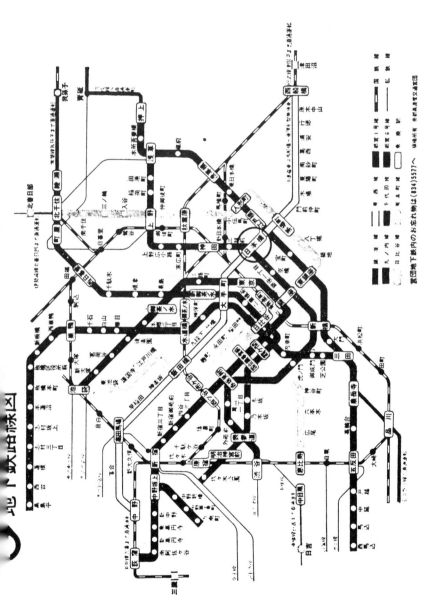

Figure 3. A contemporary network design is Chikatetsu Rosenzu, or plan of the metropolitan underground railway, Tokyo. Nihonbashi Station in east-central Tokyo (circled) stands near the point from which all distances in Japan are calculated.

9. Interactive Computer Graphics

There currently exists a great deal of interest and development in the area of graphics technology, possibly because these aspects of computer systems are becoming cost-effective for many applications. An important psychological factor is, of course, the circumstance that most people communicate more easily with pictorial and visual images than with numbers. Software and software-related packages are becoming more and more widely available commercially, and computer graphic systems are finding wide application in medicine and in research (e.g., the ACTA scanner – automatic computerized transverse-axial scanner; interactive computer graphics in nuclear medicine, pharmacology, biology, and physiology).

In a simple sense computer graphics may be defined as that technology whereby graphic or pictorial information is entered, processed, and displayed using digital computers. Most of the current work focuses on man/machine communication using cathode ray tube (CRT) consoles. A variety of unique hardware devices, including line and film plotters and CRT displays, have been designed for graphics technology (Xerox Corporation, Data Dic Inc., Proteus Display System under development by the U. S. Navy, etc.). Potential users should refer to primary literature describing and updating display technologies and new types of systems produced.

Network Designs (after Mbaeyi).

Distributing a Nation's Health Services We might consider a simple case of a housewife living in the suburbs who must go to the city to shop. While in the city she undertakes other tasks, goes to the laundry, accompanies her children to and from school. The initial figure (Figure 4) suggests an imaginary map of the community, and in the subsequent two figures the community is converted into an "ordinary graph" (Figure 5), and then into a "directed graph" (Figure 6).

We could use the same methodology to illustrate the distribution of a nation's health services. Thus we might reduce all the country's settlements to points, as depicted in Figure 7. We might then select the nation's urban centers and divide the land into r zones ($Z1, Z2 \ldots Zr$), with one urban center more or less in the middle of each zone (Figure 8). Now we may take each urban center and its accompanying zone and carve the entire district into q subzones ($SZ1, SZ2, \ldots SZq$), where q is of course any number greater than 1. Figure 9 might represent such zoning of a city by a municipal health specialist. The urban centers we might call U1, U2, etc. Assembling the country's zones, controlled by their urban centers, results in Figure 10. The final step, by which we have constructed a health network, is to join sets of remote settlements, villages, and towns to the major centers in

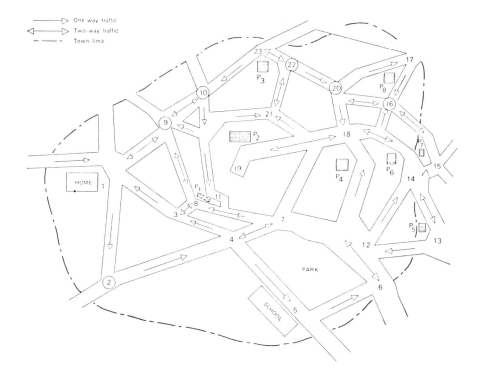

Figure 4. The housewife's community.

terms of the divisions that have been made. This results in the diagram shown as Figure 11, and the whole country is now covered with a series of networks. These networks can be interrelated and, in fact, usually are, and are controlled by a major nodal center — usually the nation's capital.

10. Computer Display of Health Data, Computer Cartography, and Computerized Mapping of Disease and Environmental Data

The value of maps as an aid in the interpretation of public health statistics has long been recognized, and there is little presently new in the concept of relating health statistics to geographic variables. A dramatic confirmation of this vital relationship can be studied in the unfolding of the story of the Burkitt lymphoma, initially recognized as a jaw tumor by Davies, and thought to be an essentially childhood disease of Ugandan Africans, rarely seen before 2 years of age, peaking between 5 and 9 years, and virtually absent after the age of 15 years. Geographic interest was heightened in the disease when it became apparent that the lymphoma

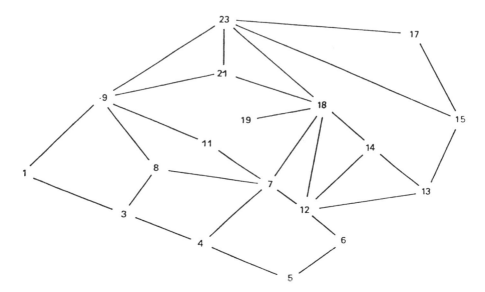

Figure 5. The community converted into an ordinary graph.

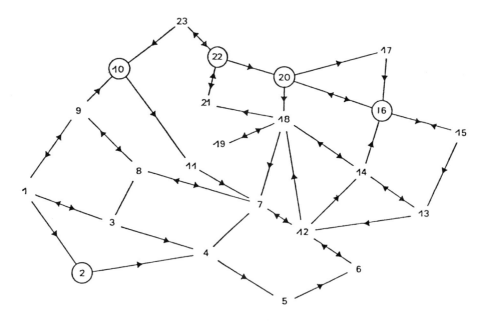

Figure 6. The community becomes a directed graph.

was also common in New Guinea, which together with tropical Africa and the Orinocco Basin formed an avifaunal region, leading to the concept that it might not be unreasonable to view this lymphoma as being due to a virus spread by an insect vector (Burkitt and Davies, 1961). This suggestion eventually led to the discovery by Epstein of the virus that bears his name.

A less exotic, but no less important, geographical relationship between disease and spatial and physical natural vectors was an empirical anticipation, years ago, of the old New England medical practitioners (as related to me by a venerable and well-worked old Maine physician). They believed that with the advent of summer and the heating up of the days, the annual increase in typhoid disease could be followed — as it traveled down the New England rivers from town to town — in a regular geographic sequence that, year by year, never varied! As the

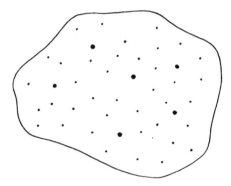

Figure 7. Schematic distribution of a country's major communities.

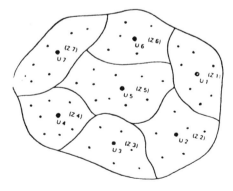

Figure 8. Symbolic designation of a country's major urban zones (U).

river waters became successively polluted, and as the heat of the summers rose, so point to point, down the river, did increasing populations of people contract the disease.

Nonetheless, coordinated structure was not given to these studies until about a decade ago. At that time the U. S. Department of Defense Advanced Research Projects Agency (ARPA) sponsored a three-year research effort into the use of computer mapping in studies of disease ecology. The case was argued by Dr. Howard Hopps, of the University of Columbia, Missouri; that because those areas in which the distribution of disease agent and host overlap mark the geographic regions where the disease can occur; evaluation of such ecologic factors as temperature, rainfall, humidity, the amount and mineral content and pH of surface water, agricultural practices, population densities of various plants and

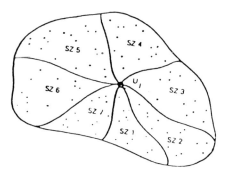

Figure 9. The jth urban zone divided into q subzones (here $q = 7$).

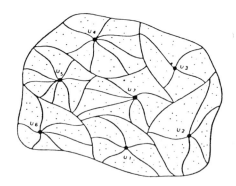

Figure 10. Zones U1 to U7 assembled as a pattern of communication.

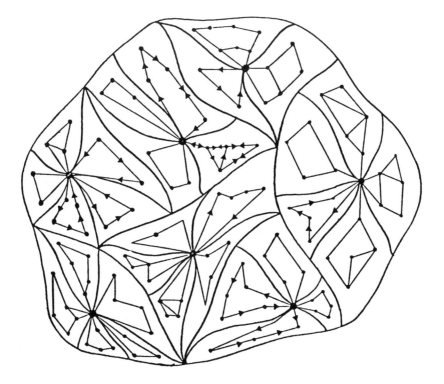

Figure 11. The resulting health-delivery network, covering entire country.

animals including man, the kinds of people involved (not only age and sex, but race, ethnic group, and tribe), and their customs − and a hundred other factors closely tied to geographic location − can help us to determine where the disease will occur, and how it will be manifest. Moreover, maps have a unique advantage over most other forms of graphic display for the general reasons that:

1. Extensive and continual usage of map forms, beginning in early childhood, has conditioned most (educated) people to an intuitive understanding of maps.
2. The map is ideally suited to a consideration of multiple factors simultaneously (e.g., place − both geographic and political − in relation to topography, population density, the location of towns and cities, the location and character of transportation routes, and the time zones.
3. Through the use of rather simple devices such as isorithms (isopleths) one can achieve a three-dimensional effect in a two-dimensional presentation

(quantity becomes the third dimension; quality and location are the other two).

Dr. Thomas Mason of the Environmental Epidemiology Branch, National Cancer Institute, has explored the manipulation and display of file data reporting deaths from cancer in the United States, and recent other group and individual efforts (Day, Gurel, Lincoln, Hyder, and Teicholz and colleagues at the Laboratory for Computer Graphics and Spatial Analysis, Harvard) have undertaken creative investigative manipulations of data methodology to analyze the potential of the variety of geographic data files that clearly are becoming available.

Programming, display, and analysis techniques useful for cartography may also be applied to other kinds of biomedical problems where results can be viewed in two dimensions plus a frequency distribution. Lincoln has suggested that flow cytofluorimetry data about tumor-cell kinetics can be analyzed in this way. A study on non-Hodgkins lymphoma has been expressed by Lincoln in terms of three-dimensional graphs, isometric plots, and slices through terrain, which can be used to characterize the proliferative behavior of cells and to subclassify tumor types.

In other areas data storage and data organizational problems that have been worked out for cartography may be applicable to this broader class of surfaces and thus transferable. Multiple-color displays can provide improved pattern recognition and discrimination. It is clear that this technology, which is still "first generation" (more advanced systems have been developed for noncivilian use), offers much promise in many other areas of medicine and health application.

11. Computer Cartography

It has been said that emphasis in information processing in the 1960s was on hardware, in the 1970s it was on software, and in the 1980s it will be on data bases. Superior methodologies must emerge as tools for accessing and interpreting increasingly voluminous amounts of data. This emerging information overload is not solely a problem for the health-related professions. Government agencies, market researchers, industrial planners, and civil and educational planners are all faced with similar problems. In a sense, our societies and our civilizations are inundated in "data," and, taking into account the extraordinary sophistication of the technologies at hand, this flood must inevitably continue to increase in the immediate future. In this view "getting the data" is by far the easiest part of any task! Our concern centers more now on how we marshal the data; how we classify, study, analyze, and integrate the data into our understanding as new knowledge; and how and by what means we may store this information.

The introduction of space satellites, for example, is instructive in these considerations. Such space systems have helped to locate one billion dollars in oil reserves and hundreds of millions of dollars in minerals, inventoried crops, estimated timber yields, monitored pollution, and studied urban sprawl, as Teicholz has noted. Prior to the launching of the first Earth Resources Technology Satellite (Landsat I) in July 1972, data gathering had been done primarily with aircraft, and essentially using cameras. Now there are three U. S. Landsats, each orbiting the earth every 103 minutes. All carry multispectral scanners and remote sensing devices, and because of their high altitude (920 kilometers or 571 miles above the surface of the earth), they are able to observe large areas at any given time – as much as 185 square kilometers of earth. Additionally their high resolution allows them to discriminate between features on the ground that are as little as 80 meters apart. Agriculture, geology, hydrology, forest and rangeland management, and marine sciences are all heirs to this information, which is captured on ultrahigh-density magnetic tape (10,000 bpi).

Yet before such information can be exploited, it must be converted into useful intelligence, corrected for errors, enhanced, classified, and interpreted. In this way, each discrete element of the picture (which is composed of thousands of tiny units known as *pixels,* each of its own unique level of brightness) is comparable to the body, which is also composed of vast numbers of cells. Analysis of the image thus gives an accounting of the state of the body. Much of this information lends itself to computer graphic representation. Yet while there has been a rapid revolution in the ability to generate data, effective use of computer-produced data has evolved much more slowly. No matter how much computer information is available, it is of no value unless it can be communicated to, and used by, a decision maker. It is in the combination of the computer's ability to generate patterns, and man's ability to interpret them, that valuable prospects for the future are found. The computer is a poor pattern recognizer. Man is a superb pattern recognizer. The combination of man and computer in prospective "data reduction" clearly has potential in computer-generated graphics and computer cartography.

Computer Cartography and Disease. Mapping of disease is by no means a new prospect. The history of many diseases has involved these concepts. Thus goiter and iodine deprivation were correlated long ago in British India by mapping villages in which the disease seemed endemic. In the long hot summers of New England, the older physicians of Maine and New Hampshire recognized each year the sequential nature of the outbreaks of typhoid in towns along the rivers from source to mouth (as noted). Yet from a perspective of Cartesian coordinates and the utilization of software modules to represent disease, the approach of geographic encoding and computer mapping of disease in medical research is but in its infancy. At the present time the technical capability exists for this goal (Day, 1978a), and some data bases are readily available from such groups as the Bureau of the Census, the federal government, and the National Cancer Institute.

Such difficulties as frequently exist are in part bound up with professional difficulty in accepting the computer, as much as with its slow introduction on grounds of cost effectiveness and usefulness in the medical and health care fields. Some of these attitudes are fortunately likely to be generational. As the older tier of medical administrators and deans depart, a younger and more intellectually vigorous second-tier generation can be anticipated who will more vigorously advance newer concepts. Historically physicians have tended to cling to the idea that they must be involved with individual patients. There is a degree of professional inhibition against thinking "in numbers." Moreover, many of the parameters relating to computer graphics and medical cartography have heretofore been quite excluded from most medical student curricula. Concepts relating to merging of different types of data, of performing statistical analyses of data and then expressing results in display files that involve spatial conceptualizations, pattern recognitions, volume, or space distribution are all "foreign." Yet it is very much in such systems for merging of data, observing changes over time, changes in the environment, life style, and so on, that much future work in the health field can be visualized.

As improved algorithms and techniques for processing and displaying spatial data improve, methods of communication and information transfer will enhance computer programming of health data. The introduction too of such methodologies as programmatic printing techniques via ink-jet color graphics produced on a raster drum plotter, a device that offers the potential of high image resolution and accuracy (Duffield, 1978), paves the way to systems in which large stores of complex data, as in medical information, can be pictorially represented. As surveillance widens our understanding in cancer research, as I have argued, geographic pathology of cancer and computer cartography of cancer data afford new possibilities of identifying cancers caused by environmental factors. Similarly, seeking computer-assisted analysis and evaluation of unusual patterns of disease that emerge from the vast pools of information that are accumulated may contribute important insights into disease profiles from people living in different geographical and cultural areas.

Allocation modelling in health care facilities planning is a field in which cartography has proved useful. Major health facilities are costly investments, and accessibility to the public is a critical factor in locating planned hospitals and clinics. Display maps can summarize evaluations of such medical facilities as, say, emergency coronary care units (CCUs). Such maps for CCUs have been evaluated in Sweden and in Massachusetts, with the goal being in both locations to determine the adequacy of the CCUs in order to identify regions not well served and to pinpoint overlarge or redundant facilities. Allocations indicated that for Massachusetts a reduction of number of CCUs (from 94 to 39) would be in order, while in Sweden additional CCUs were suggested to serve 95% of all cases within one half hour of being reported (Dutton).

In the matter of mapping diseases, because disease is almost invariably a consequence of multiple factors acting together (although not always simultaneously), strategies such as mapping of total cancer may add little to knowledge. More useful information would be anticipated from studying individual types of cancer, and investigating such factors as obstructions to cancer surveillance. Tabulation and analysis of such important data can be represented by spatial and geographic patterns, and such computer-assisted evaluations will certainly add to better understanding of the ecology of health and the causality of disease. Such programming, display, and analysis techniques as are useful for cartography may also be applied to other kinds of biomedical problems where results can be viewed in two dimensions plus a frequency distribution. Lincoln has analyzed flow cytofluorimetry data on tumor-cells kinetic in this way (as noted).

Demonstrations of important pioneering work in this area of cancer cartography, made by Professor Eric Teicholz of Harvard University, shown here, underline the dramatic potential for these new methodologies. (See Figures 12-15.)

12. Computer Medicine

Concepts that might strictly be called "computer medicine" began in the immediate post–World War II years. These early mathematical presuppositions, important as innovative and conceptual strategems, fell short of a useful clinical mark. Lipkin utilized Marginal Punched Cards for analysis of blood disease. Finally it was the research of Robert Steven Ledley and Lee B. Lusted that established the groundwork for a rational basis for computerized medicine. Their research brought forth two monographs, *Use of Computers in Biology and Medicine* (1965), by Ledley, and *Introduction to Medical Decision Making* (1968), by Lusted. Ledley, grounded in practical experience in the then-existing generation of computers, provided a mathematical background for data processing techniques. His writing on Medical Diagnosis and Medical Record Processing, as well as his observations on Special Biomedical Data Processing Methods, was devoted to the development of the groundwork for Automated Pattern Recognition, which created an avalanche in all branches of medicine. Lusted in his writings explored the practical need of scientists to employ computers in diagnostic calculations. He provided insights into the methods of computer medicine and particularly revealed to physicians how computers could serve in many ways, some of obviously superior concept in contrast to more conventional methods.

Contributions of Morris F. Collen have also been of the highest order. Since 1951 Collen has carried out investigations of the Multiphasic Screening Program at the Kaiser Research Foundation Institute in Oakland, California. Since 1963 he has examined 25,000 patients with modern electronic and automated laboratory equipment. In 1966 Collen published the operational plan of his Automatic Multitest laboratories. This included 20 stations, and the recording of all data

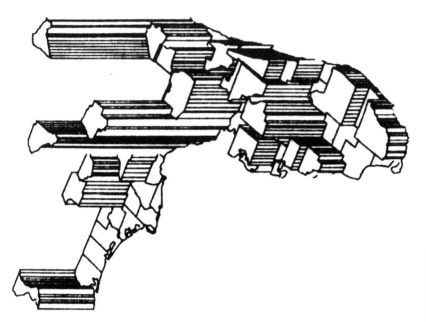

Figure 12. Counts of lip cancer from white males.

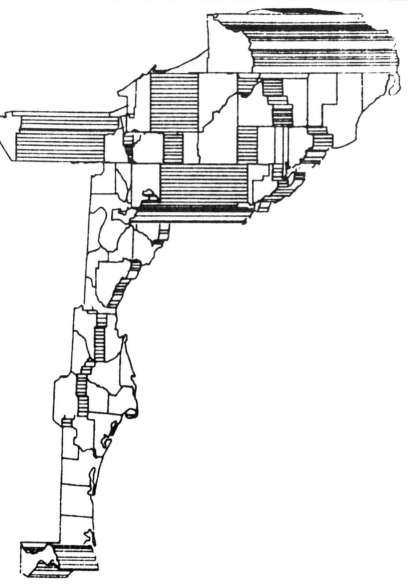

Figure 13. Rates for 100,000 population of white males, lip cancer.

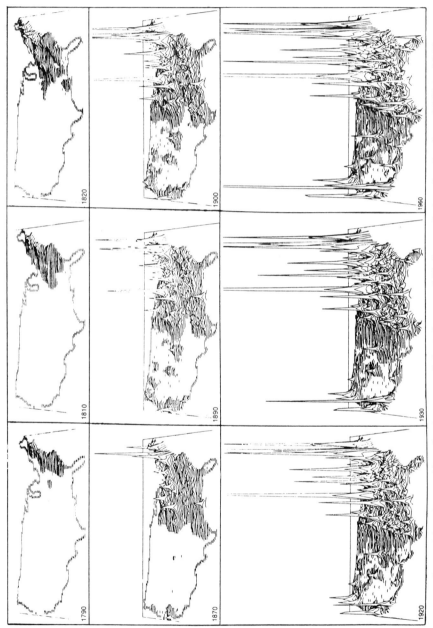

Figure 14. The manifest destiny map. Selected maps of U. S. population density from 1790 to 1960.

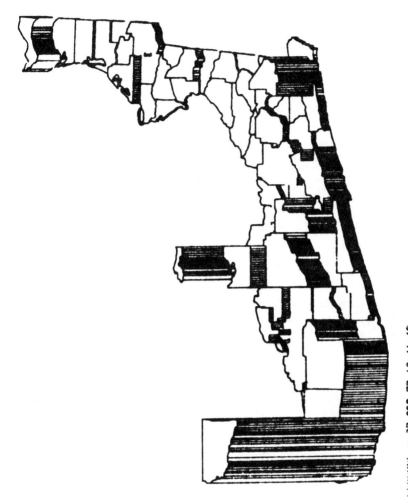

Figure 15. Counts of white female deaths from breast cancer.

on special punched cards. With his methodology and considerable experience he was able to provide firm evidence that there was:

1. Saving of patient's time through the continuous series of investigations.
2. Saving of physician's time by providing numerous findings at the initial visit.
3. Improved reliability of diagnosis based on use of automatic laboratory investigations.
4. Considerable cost reduction due to the possibility that he could obtain at least four times as many observations, at a faster rate, and at substantially the same cost.
5. Far-reaching understanding of many disease possibilities in a short time. This facilitated new diagnoses in shorter time at lower cost.
6. Through compilation of data, the facilitation of fruitful epidemiological investigations, not theretofore possible.

Such contributions as these have led to Collen's Automatic Multitest Laboratory being today a significant part of preventive medicine facilities.

The advent of automation and computers led to numerous other investigations and the utilization of electronic data processing systems in other medical work. Smith, Caceres, and Pipberger explored the cardiac field in such areas as the EKG, recordings of the cardiac heartbeat, and methodologies for improved cardiac diagnosis. H. Warner especially became well known in this work, introducing computers in the field of cardiology. Spirometry and ergometry were fully automated, and in addition numerous other procedures for the automatic evaluation of EEG, EMG, and methods for audiometric research were developed. Today in a well-run clinical chemistry laboratory, the practice of automatic indexing and computation with supervised computer control, memorization, and output, is commonplace. Such laboratories as this have effective analytical systems, run by computers, which are capable of taking over most of the functions of technical assistants.

Important also for growth in this field have been such contributions as the evolution of the Micro-scanner by Bostrom and Holcomb and the contributions of individuals such as George Wied in his *Introduction to Quantitative Cytochemistry* and his concern with automation in cytopathology. Software for this purpose was developed under the acronym TICAS (Taxonomic Intracellular Analytical System), and subsequently in several areas equipment was modified for a number of programs, including one for complete automation of differential blood analysis (Haemtrak and Lark Classifier). In a similar way, automated evaluation of X-ray photography was begun by Meyers and his collaborators in 1963 and Wood et al. in 1964, and Lodwick's parallel investigations served as an impetus for concepts of automated computation of isotope scanners.

X-ray diagnosis came to maturity through techniques of Image Reconstruction (IRC), a procedure that can in fact be traced back to procedures in the field of radioastronomy developed by Bracewell in 1956. Rosier and Klug furthered the prospect by studies on methodology of reconstruction of molecular models in the electron microscope with the aid of a series of microscopic transmissions that were received from various angles. Rowley, and Berry and Gibbs, developed techniques of image reconstruction, and in 1969 Tretiak, Eden, and Simon and in 1971 Bates and Peterson developed procedures for reconstructed tomography.

The X-ray CAT Scanner (Computer Assisted Tomography), based on pictorial reconstruction, was introduced in 1972 by Hounsfield. CAT pictures were superior, and because they were taken from different angles, afforded exceptional sharpness. Originally the CAT was used only for examination of the head but it

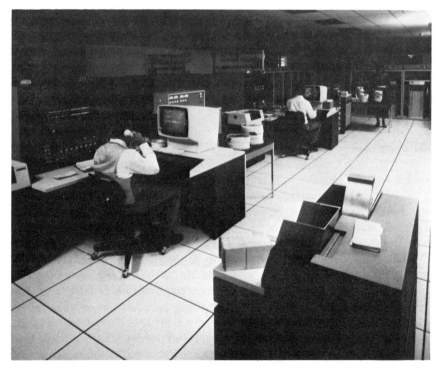

Figure 16. Data processing department. MetPath has two IBM 370/148's for the processing of all medical information for test reports. (Courtesy MetPath, New Jersey).

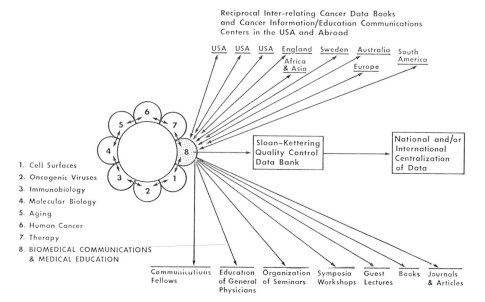

Figure 17. Information - communication computer and education model advised for Sloan Kettering Institute for Cancer Research (Day, 1974).

was later extended to the whole body by work of Ledley, Di Chiro, Luessenhop, and Twigg.

Reflection on these improvements emphasizes the understanding that the body scanner is dependent not only on the use of the detector and computer, but that it must utilize important software to enable visualization of the pictures — such essential programs as Bach Projection, Iterative Reconstruction, Analytic Reconstruction, Magnification of Contrast, Filtration, Smoothing, and so on, have all added to improvements in the operational procedures.

While the body scanner may appear to be the newest development of computer medicine, further enormous strides are being made. Progress is being made toward the development of minicomputers. The time is not far off, conceivably, when every practicing physician will be using his own console in consultation via computer-based data resources toward solution and establishment of disease description and diagnosis. Computer medicine is as realistic as is the time-honored stethoscope assistance toward a reliable diagnosis for the ill patient.

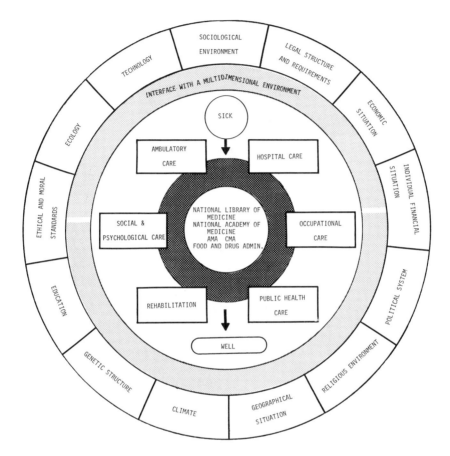

Figure 18.   Concept of master plan for medical/health information network. (Source: P. L. Reichertz: "Hospital and Health Care Systems," Boston/Cambridge, Mass., 1975.)

LITERATURE AND SOURCES

Hogben, Lancelot: *Mathematics For The Millions.* London: George Allen and Unwin Ltd, 1942.

Jaglom, A. M., and Jaglom, I.: *Wahrscheinlichkeit and Information.* Berlin: VEB Deutscher Verlag der Wissenschafter, 1960.

Jaki, Stanley L.: *Brain, Mind and Computers.* New York: Herder and Herder, 1969.

King, Linda S.: "The Future of Chemical Information." In *Communication of Scientific Information* (ed. by Stacey B. Day), pp. 149–58. Basel: Karger, 1975.

Kolmogorow, A. N.: "Arbeitzen zur Informationstheorie." In *Mathematische Forschungsberichte.* Berlin: VEB Deutscher Verlag der Wissenschaften, 1960.

Mbaeyi, Peter: N. O.: "An Operational Model to Distribute A Nation's Health Services." *Impact. UNESCO.* 26(4):277–90, 1976.

Mbaeyi, Peter: N. O.: Networks. Personal discussions. 1978.

McCulloch, I. W. S.: "The Design of Machines To Simulate The Behavior of the Human Brain." In *IRE National Convention.* Symposium. New York, 1955.

Pollack, Seymour V.: *A Guide to Fortran IV.* New York and London: Columbia University Press, 1965.

Rothman, Stanley, and Mosmann, Charles: *Computers and Society.* S.R.A. 1972.

Shannon, C. E., and Weaver, W.: *The Mathematical Theory of Communication.* Urbana: University of Illinois Press, 1963.

Sherman, Herbert: Introduction to English translastion by Vishnevskiy (op. cit.). Lexington, Massachusetts: M.I.T. Lincoln Laboratory. 1974.

Shipton, Harold, W.: "Memory For Computers." In *Communication of Scientific Information* (ed. by Day), pp. 184–93. Basel: Karger, 1975.

Turing, A. M.: "Computing Machinery and Intelligence." *Mind* 59:433–60, 1950.

Turing, A. M.: "Can A Machine Think?" In *The World of Mathematics* (ed. by James R. Newman). New York: Simon and Schuster, Inc., 1956.

Weiner, Norbert: "Some Moral and Technical Consequences of Automation." *Science* 131:1357, 1960.

Weiner, Norbert: *Cybernetics or Control and Communication in the Animal and the Machine.* New York: John Wiley and Sons, Inc., 1961.

Unger, G.: *Cybernetics and Man's Responsibility for His Consciousness.* Mathematisch–Physikalisches Institut. CH-4143. Dornach, Schweiz.

Vishnevskiy, A. A., Artobolevskiy, I. I., and Bykhovskiy, M. L.: *Machine Diagnosis and Information Retrieval in Medicine in the U.S.S.R.*, 1973. Translated and presented as DHEW Publication No. (NIH) 73-424.

Other Sources

Altman, P. L.; Challinor, D.; and Marcy, W. see respective chapters in *Communication of Scientific Information,* edited by Stacey B. Day, S. Karger, Basel, Switzerland, 1975.

Studies of Langer and Brandej, Gorry, and others, see Section on Biosocial Development and Biosciences Communications, *Volume 1, Companion To The Life Sciences,* edited by Stacey B. Day, Van Nostrand Reinhold, New York, 1979.

For discussions on Leach, Bishoff, Price, and others see *Health Communications,* By Stacey B. Day, a publication of the International Foundation For Biosocial Development And Human Health, New York, 1979. Other background reading is available in *Biopsychosocial Health,* edited by Stacey B. Day, International Foundation For Biosocial Development And Human Health, New York, 1980.

NOTES

Computer Cartography and Computer Modelling of Data

For discussions on geographic pathology of disease see, e.g., J. N. P. Davies, Concept of Cancer or Concept of Cancers, *Laval Medical,* Vol. 39, January 1968; J. N. P. Davies and N. J. Vianna, Epidemiological Evidence of the Role of Viruses in Human Cancer with Special Reference to Lymphomas, in *Characterization of Human Tumors,* International Congress Series No. 321 (*Proceedings*, Bologna, April 4-6, 1973); and Hopps, Howard et al.: *Computerized Mapping Disease and Environmental Data,* Army Research Office Publication, 1968.

For computer modelling see summary and extension remarks of seminar group on Computer Modelling and Cancer Data, New York City, 24/4/1977, published in *Companion To The Life Sciences,* Vol. I, Van Nostrand Reinhold, New York, 1978 (Stacey B. Day; Howard C. Hopps; Okan Gurel; S. S. Hyder; Eric Teicholz; and T. Lincoln).

Also see Eric Teicholz and Mark Hanson, Computer Display of Cancer Data, *Biosciences Communications* 5:155-164, 1979 (Health Communications and Informatics).

See also J. T. Mason, F. W. McKay, R. Hoover, W. J. Blot, and J. F. Fraumeni. *Atlas of Cancer Mortality for U. S. Counties 1950-1969,* DHEW Publication No. (NIH) 75-780.

Epistemology of Medical/Health Information Systems: Definition of Some Useful Terms

Epistemology — is the theory of the basis and methods of knowledge.

Inquirer — is an end-user of a system. He/she can be classified as a "type" when he/she becomes locked into his/her way of perception of the global (world systems) through a fixed approach. These are basically four types of inquirers: (a) mathematical, (b) realist, (c) intuitive, and (d) conflictual type.

Inquiring system — has the purpose of creating knowledge, which means:

1. One is creating the capability of choosing the right means for one's desired ends.
2. The measure of performance is to be defined as "inquiring level of the scientific and educational excellence of all society," a measure yet to be developed.
3. The client is mankind; i.e., all humans should gain.
4. Other components have the disciplines, but the design of inquiry along esoteric, disciplinary lines is probably wrong.

5. The environment of inquiring systems is a very critical aspect of the design.

Inquiry — is an activity that produces knowledge.

Machine era — is an era in which parts of a system were viewed and explained separately without an understanding of the whole.

Postindustrial society — is a society in which industrial productivity is no longer the dominant economic activity.

Quasi-systems — are systems designed on the present notions of the industrial society.

Systems approach — is a process based on viewing a problem as a set of inter-related, independent parts that work together for the overall objective of the whole.

Systems era — is an era in which instead of explaining a whole in terms of its parts, parts begin to be explained in terms of the whole. Therefore, the things that are to be analyzed are viewed as parts of the larger wholes rather than as wholes to be taken apart.

Systems science — is an amalgamation of all parts of sciences into an integral whole. Thus, systems science is not a science but a science taken as whole and applied to the study of a whole.

Systems theory — is an attempt to assess the impact of the human thought processes on the systems science. On one hand the basis for investigation are styles of agreement–summarization (e.g., Platonian vs. Aristotelian style). On the other hand, the basic understanding rests in the nature of the inquirer.

SIMPLE GLOSSARY OF GENERAL-PURPOSE COMPUTER LANGUAGE

This glossary presents a few of the common terms associated with the general subject of computers and the life sciences. The list is not to be considered as anything other than a simple guide that may help to amplify some of the discussions in this chapter.

Access: Related to memory device. Core memory is called *random access* when any word can be obtained at any time without regard to its serial order. Drum, tape, and disc memories are *serial access.*

Algol: ALGOrithmic language of an algebraic family similar to FORTRAN. Popular in Europe, but less so in the United States. The Association for Computing Machinery uses ALGOL as a publication language for computer algorithms published in its journals.

Algorithm: A precisely specified method for providing a solution to a problem. An algorithm is not a program, because it is not written expressly for a particular computing device that is to be used.

Binary number: The binary system uses the concepts of absolute value and positional value in the same way as the decimal. The binary system uses only two absolute values, zero and one, and the positional values are powers of 2. The following table demonstrates the correspondence between decimal and binary numbers as shown:

Decimal	Binary
0	0
1	1
2	10
3	11
4	100
5	101
6	110
7	111
8	1000

Bit: Basic unit of information in a digital computer's logic or memory.

Boolian algebra: Mathematical basis proposed by George Boole for the manipulation of an operation with classes, sets, and logical elements. It is a tool in computer hardware design.

Byte: Group of bits needed to produce a single unique character of information. Digital processors now use eight-bit bytes.

Computer: A machine for performing complex processes on information without manual intervention. *Analog computers* perform this function by directly measuring and transforming continuous physical quantities such as electrical voltage. *Digital computers* represent numerical quantities that can be manipulated logically by discrete electrical states.

Console (often called terminal or display): Device with which humans communicate with machine system, usually computer. Devices include portable terminals that can be attached to any telephone line, typewriter keyboards modified to put out coded electrical signals representing the keys struck, or other forms of electric signals that cause type bars to move and characters to appear on paper. Audible codes may be transmitted via the telephone system which can convert the audible signal into an electrical pattern and send it to a computer. Interactive display consoles (e.g., a surveillance officer studying a radar return) incorporate the principle of the cathode ray tube (CRT) in the display console. The cathode ray tube is, in principle, the same device that is used in the home television set. A light pen may be used to interact with a computer. The console is thus part of the central processor from which the computing system is operated and monitored.

Core memory: The memory of most modern computers is made up of magnetic cores, a core being a tiny ring of ferromagnetic material that can be magnetized in either a clockwise or counterclockwise direction. These magnetized components store information by virtue of combinations of magentization direction as instructed by the digital computer via its circuitry.

Data: Information, coded or uncoded, numeric or nonnumeric.

Data base: An integrated file of data used by many processing applications.

Electronic data processing machines (E.D.P. or processors): Digital computers are sometimes referred to as processors or electronic data processing machines. To distinguish the physical equipment from the programs such machines are frequently called *hardware.*

Keypunch: An input device by which an operator is able to transfer information into the computer. Commonly the information is translated from its original form (handwritten, typed, or printed document, etc.), by such techniques as those utilizing a typewriter to punch holes.

Input/output: Generalized terms for the techniques, devices, or strategies used to communicate with data processing equipment and for the data involved in these communications. Often known as I/O.

Logic: In computers, circuitry required for implementation of instructions to enable machine to carry out its task. The manner in which the network of switching and memory devices is organized is called *machine logic.* The physical basis for these elements consists of the actual electronic components of which the machine is constructed.

Program: Sequential instructions encoded in computer language for the performance of a given task on command.

Software: Programs and other logical structures that enable computer hardware to problem-solve.

SELECTED BIBLIOGRAPHY

Abbott, C. E.: "Computer-Assisted System in a Multi-Specialty Clinic in Manitoba — Phase I." Symposium on Medical Informatics, Toulouse, France, March 1978.

"Ambulatory Medical Records — Uniform Basic Data Set." Department of Health, Education and Welfare, Publication No. (HRA) 75-1453, Series 4, No. 16, Superintendent of Documents, Washington, D. C., 1974.

Anderson, H. O.: "First Step in the Development of a Hospital EDP System." Medinfo 1974 *Proceedings.* Amsterdam: North-Holland Publishing Company, 1975.

Anderson, J., and J. Beer Gabel: "Conclusion on Systems Life Cycle." *Proceedings,* Working Conference on Information Systems for Patient Care, 1975. Amsterdam: North-Holland Publishing Company, 1976.

Anderson, J., and J. M. Forsythe: Medinfo 1974 *Proceedings.* Amsterdam: North-Holland Publishing Company, 1975.

Anderson, J., F. Gremy, and J. C. Pages: "Education in Informatics of Health Personnel." Amsterdam: North-Holland Publishing Company, 1974.

Aronsson, T., et al.: "A Data System for Clinical Chemistry Laboratories — Considerations, Brief Description and Evaluation." Medinfo 1974 *Proceedings*. Amsterdam: North-Holland Publishing Company, 1975.

Atsumi, K.: "Technological and Social Assessment on Medical Information Systems." *Proceedings,* Information Systems For Patient Care, 1975. Amsterdam: North-Holland Publishing Company, 1976.

Bakker, A. R.: "The Information System of Leiden University Hospital." *Proceedings,* Information Systems For Patient Care, 1975. Amsterdam: North-Holland Publishing Company, 1976.

Bancsich, J.: "Wielab — A New Hardware Concept and its Related Software Support for Automatic Sample Identification and Conversational Output in Clinical Laboratories." Medinfo 1974 *Proceedings*. Amsterdam: North-Holland Publishing Company, 1975.

Barber, B.: "The Approach to an Evaluation of the London Hospital Computer Project." Medinfo 1974 *Proceedings*. Amsterdam: North-Holland Publishing Company, 1975.

Barnet, O.: Director. Costar: Computer Stored Ambulatory Record. Laboratory of Computer Sciences, Massachusetts General Hospital, Boston, Massachusetts, 1977.

Barnett, G. O.: "Costar: A Progress Report." Laboratory of Computer Sciences, Boston, Massachusetts, Massachusetts General Hospital, 1975.

Barnett, G. O., et al.: "The Role of Feedback in Quality Assurance — An Application of Computer Based Ambulatory Medical Information System." *Proceedings,* Conference on Assessing Physician Performance in Ambulatory Care. American Society of Internal Medicine, 1976.

Beaumont, J. O.: "Intensive Care." Medinfo 1974 *Proceedings*. Amsterdam: North-Holland Publishing Company, 1975.

Bernholtz, B., F. B. Filis, et al.: "Proposal for a Joint Research and Development Program by the Department of Family and Community Medicine and Industrial Engineering to Develop and Implement and Improved Family and Community Medicine." Mimeograph, Toronto: University of Toronto, 1975.

Berry, M. V., and D. F. Gibbs: "The Interpretation of Optical Projections." *Proc. R. Soc. A* 314:143–52, 1969.

Blois, M. S., and A. I. Wasserman: "A Graduate Program in Medical Information Science." Medinfo 1974 *Proceedings*. Amsterdam: North-Holland Publishing Company, 1975.

Blois, M. S., and A. I. Wasserman: "The Integration of Hospital Information Services." *Proceedings,* Information Systems for Patient Care, 1975. Amsterdam: North-Holland Publishing Company, 1976.

Bohm, K.: "Protection and Confidentiality of Medical Data." Medinfo 1974 *Proceedings*. Amsterdam: North-Holland Publishing Company, 1975.

Bolt, Beranek and Newman, Inc.: "The CAPO Project — Evaluation of an Automated Medical History in Office Practice." Report 2471. Cambridge, Massachusetts, 1972.

Bolt, M. C., J. Box, C. R. Evans, and J. Wilson: "An Investigation of Computer Administration of a Psychological Test to Psychiatric Patients." *Proceedings,*

Information Systems for Patient Care, 1975. Amsterdam: North-Holland Publishing Company, 1976.

Boraas, B. A.: "Efficacy of Computer Related Services Within a Health Sciences Center." Medinfo 1974 *Proceedings*. Amsterdam: North-Holland Publishing Company, 1975.

Bostrom, R. C., and W. G. Holcomb: "A Digital Screening Cytophotometer." *IEEE Int. Conv. Record* 9:110–19, 1963.

Bracewell, R. N.: "Strip Integration in Radio Astronomy." *Aust. J. Phys.* 9:198–217, 1956.

Brandejs, J. F.: *Health Informatics*. Amsterdam: North-Holland Publishing Company, 1976.

Brandejs, J. F.: *Medical Records of the Future*. Canadian Medical Association, SS&ER (Unit), 1978a. Ottawa.

Brandejs, J. F.: *Physician's Primer on Computers: Private Practice*. Lexington, Massachusetts: Lexington Books, 1978b.

Brandejs, J. F., et al.: "Information Systems, Parts I–VII." *Can. Med. Assoc. J.* No 113, 1975.

Brandejs, J. F., G. C. Pace, and W. Cara: *Basic Computer-Aided Physician Office (C.A.P.O.) Handbook*. CMA, Ottawa, 1977.

Brodman, K., and A. J. van Woerkom: "Computer-Aided Diagnostic Screening for 100 Common Diseases." *J.A.M.A.* 197:901–5, 1966.

Brodman, K., and A. van Woerkom: "Computer Aided Diagnostic Screening for 100 Common Diseases." *Proceedings, Information Systems for Patient Care, 1975*. Amsterdam: North-Holland Publishing Company, 1976.

Brodman, K., A. J. Erdmann, I. Lorge, and H. G. Wolff: "The Cornell Medical Index: An Adjunct to Medical Interview." *J.A.M.A.* 140:530–34, 1949.

Brodman, K., A. J. Erdmann, I. Lorge, and H. G. Wolff: "The Cornell Medical Index–Health Questionnaire, II. As a Diagnostic Instrument." *J.A.M.A.* 145:152–57, 1951.

Brodman, K., A. J. van Woerkom, A. J. Erdmann, and L. Goldstein: "Interpretation of Symptoms with a Data-Processing Machine." *Arch. Intern. Med.* 103:776–82, 1959.

Broman, S.: "Structuring Information for Computer Aided Evaluation of Methods and Results of Medical Care." Medinfo 1974 *Proceedings*. Amsterdam: North-Holland Publishing Company, 1975.

Bross, I. D. J., et al.: "Feasibility of Automated Information Systems in the User's Natural Language." *Am. Sci.* 57(2):193–205, 1969.

de Bruijn, W. K.: "A National Hospital Automation Plan for the Netherlands." Medinfo 1974 *Proceedings*. Amsterdam: North-Holland Publishing Company, 1975.

von Brunt, E.: "The Kaiser Permanente Medical Information System." *Proceedings, Conference on Medical Information Systems*. San Francisco, 1970.

von Brunt, E. E., L. S. Davis, et al.: "The Kaiser Permanente Pilot Medical Data System." *Proceedings, Conference on Health Technology Systems*. San Francisco, 1973.

von Brunt, E. E., L. S. Davis, J. F. Terdiman, and M. F. Collen: "The Kaiser Permanente Hospital Computer System." In *Hospital Computer Systems* (ed. by M. F. Collen). New York: John Wiley and Sons, 1974.

Bryans, A. M., G. A. Southall, L. S. Valberg, J. J. Waldron, B. Valberg, and A. S. Kraus: "A New Type of Facility in Medical Education: The Clinical Learning Centre." *J. Med. Ed.* 50:277–84, 1975.

Budd, M. A., and B. Reiffen: "Implications of Computer Science for Developing Ambulatory Medical Record Systems." *Med. Care* 11(2):132–37, 1973.

Cass, William, et al.: "Development of a Computer-Based Medical Record System." *Proceedings,* Fifth Annual Conference of the Society for Computer Medicine, 1975.

Castleman, P. A., P. Bertoni, and S. Whitehead: "An Ambulatory Care Center Support System." *Proceedings,* Information Systems for Patient Care, 1975. Amsterdam: North-Holland Publishing Company, 1976.

van Cauwenberge H., A. M. Gyselynck, and G. Rorive: "Computer Assistance to Medical Care and General Organization in a Dialysis System." XI Congress of the European Dialysis and Transplant Association. Tel Aviv, Israel, November 3–8, 1974.

CHA (Canadian Hospital Association): "The National Symposium on Computer Applications in the Health Field." Papers. Ottawa, 1970.

Chamberlin, D. D.: "Relational Data Base Management Systems." *Computing Surveys* 8(1):43–66, March 1976.

Chouinard, J. L.: "The Future of Computers in Canadian Health Care." *Proceedings*, DPI/CIPS Conference. Ottawa, June 1974.

Cohen, S. N., et al.: "Computer Based Monitoring and Reporting of Drug Interaction." Medinfo 1974 *Proceedings.* Amsterdam: North-Holland Publishing Company, 1975.

Collen, M. F.: "Machine Diagnosis from a Multiphasic Screening Program." 5th IBM Medical Symposium. Endicott, New York, October 7, 1963.

Collen, M. F.: "Computers in Preventive Health Services Research." 7th IBM Medical Symposium. Poughkeepsie, New York, October 27, 1965.

Collen, M.: "Periodic Health Examinations Using an Automated Multitest Laboratory." *J.A.M.A.* 195:830–33, 1966.

Collen, M. F.: "General Requirements for a Medical Information System (MIS)." *Computers Biomed. Res.* 3:393–406, 1970.

Collen, M. F. (ed.): *Hospital Computer Systems.* New York: John Wiley and Sons, 1974.

Collen, M. F.: "Self-Administered Questionnaire." *J. Clin. Computing* 7(1): 1977.

Collen, M. F. (ed.): *Multiphasic Health Testing Services.* New York: John Wiley and Sons, 1977.

Collen, M. F., and L. S. Davis: "The Multitest Laboratory in Health Care." *J. Occup. Med.* Vol. 2, No. 7, 1969.

Collen, M. F., J. F. Cutler, A. B. Siegelaub, and R. L. Cella: "Reliability of a Self-Administered Medical Questionnaire." *Arch. Intern. Med.* 23:664–81, 1969.

Collen, M. F., P. H. Kidd, R. Feldman, and J. L. Cutler: "Cost Analysis of a Multiphasic Screening Program." *New Engl. J. Med.* 280(19):1043–50, 1969.

Collen, M. F., L. S. Davis, and E. E. van Brunt: "The Computer Medical Record in Health Screening." *Meth. Infor. Med.* 10:138–42, 1971.

Collen, M. F., L. S. Davis, E. E. von Brunt, and J. F. Terdiman: "Functional Goals and Problems in Large Scale Patient Record Management and Automated Screening." FASEB Conference on the Computer as a Research Tool in the Life Sciences. Aspen, Colorado, June 1974.

Cormack, A. M.: "Representation of a Function by Its Line Integrals with Some Radiological Applications." *J. Appl. Phys.* 34:2722, 1963.

Cormack, A. M.: "Representation of a Function by Its Line Intergrals with Some Radiological Applications. II." *J. Appl. Phys.* 35:2908–13, 1964.

Covvey, H. D., and N. H. McAlister: "Data Into Information: The Electronic Philospher's Stone." *Can. Med. Assoc. J.* 115:358–59, 1976.

Covvey, H. D., and N. H. McAlister: "Conspicuous Computing; If there Are Users There Must be Pushers." *Can. Med. Assoc. J.* 116:183–87, 1977.

Crawford, D.: "Measurement of the Effectiveness of On-Line Biomedical Computing in Multiphasic Health Testing." *J. Assoc. Adv. Med. Instru.* 6(1) 1972.

Curran, W. J., et al.: "Privacy, Confidentiality and Other Legal Considerations in the Establishment of a Centralized Health Data System." *New Engl. J. Med.* Vol. 281, No. 241, 1969.

Daechsel, W. F. O., and E. Clemence: "Computers in the Kitchen." *Can. Hosp.,* pp. 34–36, June 1973.

Davis, L. S.: "Prototype for Future Computer Medical Records." *Computers Biomed. Res.* 3:539–54, 1970.

Davis, L. S.: "Problems Facing Large Health Information Systems." Medical *Proceedings.* Atlanta, August 1973.

Davis, L. S.: "A System Approach to Medical Information." *Meth. Infor. Med.* 12:1–6, 1973.

Davis, L. S., and L. N. Bell: "Distributed Medical Data Base Configurations." *Proceedings,* 4th Annual Conference on Society for Computer Medicine, Clinical Medicine and the Computer. New Orleans, November 1974.

Davis, L. S., and T. A. Simacek: "Distributed Data Base Medical Information Systems." *Proceedings,* Information Systems for Patient Care, 1975. Amsterdam: North-Holland Publishing Company, 1976.

Davis, L. S., M. F. Collen, L. Rubin, and E. E. von Brunt: "Computer Stored Medical Record." *Computers Biomed. Res.* 1:452–69, 1968.

Day, Stacey B.: "Georgraphic Pathology of Cancer and Computer Cartography of Cancer Data." In *A Companion to the Life Sciences,* Vol. I (ed. by Stacey B. Day), pp. 270–77. New York: Van Nostrand Reinhold, 1978.

Day, Stacey B.: "Moderator's Remarks, Session on Medical Cartography: Its Applications in Public Health." Harvard Computer Graphics Conference on Computer Mapping Software and Data Bases, Application and Dissemination. Cambridge, Massachusetts, July 1978.

Day, Stacey B., and E. Teicholz: "Computer Graphics: Application of Computer Graphics in Medicine and Health Care Sciences." Special monograph issue, *Biosci. Commun.* 1:257–347, 1975. 41 figures.

Deland, E. C., and B. D. Waxman: *Review of Hospital Information Systems.* Santa Monica, California: The Rand Corporation, 1970.

DeRosier, D. J., and A. Klug: "Reconstruction of Three Dimensional Structures from Electron Micrographs." *Nature (London)* 217:130–34, 1968.

Dixon, P. J.: "Communications Between Hospitals and Family Doctors." Medinfo 1974 *Proceedings.* Amsterdam: North-Holland Publishing Company, 1975.

Duffield, Peter L.: "Ink-jet Color Graphics." Presented at the SPSE Annual Meeting. Washington, D.C., May 1978.

van Egmond, J., et al.: "Belgium Interuniversity Project on Computerization of the Medical Record Supported by the Belgian Government." Medinfo 1974 *Proceedings.* Amsterdam: North-Holland Publishing Company, 1975.

van Egmond, J., L. Decoussemaker, R. J. Wieme, and W. Bossaert: "Implementation of an Information System for Patient Care in the University Hospital of Gent." *Proceedings*, Information Systems for Patient Care, 1975. Amsterdam: North-Holland Publishing Company, 1976.

Elfquist, B.: "A Patient Scheduling System." Medinfo 1974 *Proceedings.* Amsterdam: North-Holland Publishing Company, 1975.

Ericsson, O., W. Schneider, and K. Vogel: "The Problem of Privacy in a Computer Based Integrated Health Care Information System." Medinfo 1974 *Proceedings.* Amsterdam: North-Holland Publishing Company, 1975.

Evans, C., and H. R. Price: "The Doctor Patient Interaction or Consultation. Can the Computer Assist in This Dialogue?" *Proceedings,* Information Systems for Patient Care, 1975. Amsterdam: North-Holland Publishing Company, 1976.

Evans, C. R., H. C. Price, and J. Wilson: "Computer Interrogation of Patients with Respiratory Complaints in a London Hospital." 1973.

Farley, E. S.: "An Integrated System for the Recording and Retrieval of Medical Data in Primary Care Setting." Eight articles in *J. Fam. Pract.* 1974.

Gabrieli, E. R.: Editor in Chief, *J. Clin. Computing,* Vol. 1–7, 1971–78.

Goldberg, M., A. G. Greenburg, D. J. Werner, L. M. Nyhus, and G. K. Krulee: "Medical Summaries Revisted: The Design Problem." *Proceedings,* San Diego Bio-Medical Symposium, p. 192. 1973.

Goldberg, M., D. J. Werner and A. G. Greenburg: "Designing Computerized Medical Information Systems Through Simulation." *Proceedings,* 7th Annual Simulation Symposium, p. 97. Tampa, Florida, 1974.

Greenburg, A. G.: "The Role of the Computer in Patient Care." Chapter 4 in *Surgery Annual,* Vol. 6 (ed. by L. M. Nyhus). New York: Appleton-Century-Croft, 1974.

Griesser, G.: "Presentation and Use of Medical Basic Information in Kiel KIS." *Proceedings,* Information Systems for Patient Care, 1975. Amsterdam: North-Holland Publishing Company, 1976.

Grossman, J. H., et al.: "An Automated Medical Record System." *J.A.M.A.* 224:1616–21, 1973.

Haessler, H. A., T. Holland, and E. L. Elshtain: "Evolution of an Automated Data Base History." *Arch. Intern. Med.* 134:586–91, 1974.

Hall, D. L., G. S. Lodwick, R. Kruger, and S. J. Dwyer: "Computer Diagnosis of Heart Disease." *Radiol. Clin. N. Am.* 9:533–541, 1971.

Hall, D. L., G. S. Lodwick, R. P. Kruger, S. J. Dwyer, and J. R. Townes: "Direct Computer Diagnosis of Rheumatic Heart Disease." *Radiology* 101:497–509, 1971.

Hannah, K. J.: "The Relationship Between Nursing and Medical Informatics in Community Health Care Settings." Medinfo 77 *Proceedings.* Amsterdam: North-Holland Publishing Company, 1977.

Hawkins, R. B.: "Introduction of a User-Oriented H.I.S. Into a Community Hospital Setting: Introductory Agents and Their Roles." Medinfo 1974 *Proceedings.* Amsterdam: North-Holland Publishing Company, 1975.

Hayes, J. E., Jr.: "The Medical Information System (MIS) of 1975." *Computers Biomed. Res.* 3:555–60, 1970.

Health Computer Information Bureau. *Health Computer Application in Canada.* Catalogue and descriptions, Vols. 1–3. Ottawa: HCIB, 1974–76.

Heisterkamp, Charles, III: "A Complete Minicomputer System for the Physician's Office." Medinfo 77 *Proceedings.* Amsterdam: North-Holland Publishing Company, 1977.

Henley, R. R., G. Widerhold, et al.: *An Analysis of Automated Ambulatory Medical Record Systems,* Vol. 1: *Findings,* Vol. 2: *Background,* San Francisco Medical Center, University of California, 1975. National Technical Information Service, U. S. Department of Commerce, Springfield, Virginia 22151 as PB 254234.

Holland, B., P. M. Holland, and R. Hsieh: "Automated Multiphasic Health Testing." *Public Health Rep.* 90(2):133–39, March–April 1975.

Hounsfield, G. N.: British patent no. 1283915 (1972).

Hounsfield, G. N.: "Computerized Transverse Axial Scanning (Tomography). Part 1. Description of System." *Br. J. Radiol.* 46:1016–22, 1973.

Hyde, C. M., and R. E. Smith: "Computer Applications in Cardiology." IBM World Trade Customer Seminar. Eurpoean Education Centre, Blaricom, The Netherlands, October 6–8, 1965.

Jarcho, S.: "Morgagni and Auenbrugger in the Retrospect of Two Hundred Years." *Bull. Hist. Med.* 35:489–96, 1961.

Klingenmaier, C. H., P. R. Moyer, J. I. Aunon, M. J. Shaffer, F. A. Siegel, and J. C. Rios: "A Method of Computers-Assisted Pacemaker Surveillance from a Patient's Home via Telephone." *Computers Biomed. Res.* 6:327–35, 1973.

Knight, J. E., and J. Streeter: "The Computer as an Aid to Nursing Records." *Nursing Times,* pp. 233–35, February 19, 1970.

Knight, R. M., and S. J. Cunningham: "Automated Pediatric Interview and Educational Assessment." Medinfo 77 *Proceedings.* Amsterdam: North-Holland Publishing Company, 1977.

Kuhl, D. E., and R. Q. Edwards: "Image Separation Radioisotope Scanning." *Radiology* 80:653–61, 1963.

Ledley, R. S.: *Use of Computers in Biology and Medicine.* New York: McGraw-Hill, 1965.

Ledley, R. S.: "High Speed Automatic Analysis of Biomedical Pictures." *Science* 146:216–23, 1964.

Ledley, R. S., G. Di Chiro, A. J. Luessenhop, and H. L. Twigg: "Computerized X-ray Tomography of the Human Body." *Science* 186:207–12, 1974.

Lincoln, Thomas L., and Stanley E. Shackney: "Computer Graphics in the Interpretation of Cell Kinetics." Presented at the Harvard Computer Graphics Conference on Computer Mapping Software and Data Bases: Applications and Dissemination. Cambridge, Massachusetts, July 1978.

Lipkin, L. E., W. C. Watt, and R. A. Kirsch,: "The Analysis, Synthesis and Description of Biological Images." *Ann. N. Y. Acad. Sci.* 128:984–1012, 1966.

Lipkin, M.: "The Role of Data Processing in the Diagnostic Process." Conference *Proceedings*, The Diagnostic Process. University of Michigan, May 9–11, 1968.

Lipkin, M., and J. Hardy: "Medical Correlation of Data in Differential Diagnosis of Hematological Diseases." *J.A.M.A.* 166:113–125, 1958.

Lodwick, G. S.: "A Probabilistic Approach to the Diagnosis of Bone Tumors." *Radiol. Clin. N. Am.* 3:479–487, 1965.

Lodwick, G. S., A. H. Turner, L. B. Lusted, and A. W. Templeton: "Computer-Aided Analysis of Radiographic Images." *J. Chron. Dis.* 19:485–96, 1966.

Lurie, R. S.: "COSTAR — Cost and Benefits." *Proceedings of the 1974 MUMPS Users' Group Meeting,* pp. 140–45. St. Louis, Missouri: MUMPS Users' Group, 1974.

Lusted, L. B.: *Introduction to Medical Decision Making.* Springfield, Illinois: Charles C. Thomas, 1968.

Lyman, M.: "Experience with the Automated Medical Record System at the Bellevue Pediatric Clinic." *Proceedings,* Third Illinois Conference on Medical Information Systems. Department of Information Engineering, University of Illinois, Chicago, Illinois, 1976.

McDonald, D. J.: "Use of a Computer to Detect and Respond to Clinical Events: Its Effect on Clinician Behavior." *Ann. Intern. Med.* 84:162–67, 1976.

McFarlane, A. H., G. R. Norman, W. O. Spitzer, and G. C. Abbot: *Computerized Ambulatory Patient Records* Documentation Vols. I, II, and and III. Department of Family Medicine, McMaster University, Hamilton, Ontario. 1976.

McLendor, S.: "Clinical Laboratory Automation and Data Processing." *Med. Instru.* 8(5): September 1974.

McQuitty, G. D. H.: "An Account of the Development and First Three Years Experience in Running a Primary Care Data Base." Medinfo 77 *Proceedings.* Amsterdam: North-Holland Publishing Company, 1977.

Meddings, E., and P. Foley: "Development of a Computer Based Information System for Cumulative Patient Profiles in a Family Practice Setting." Medinfo 77 *Proceedings.* Amsterdam: North-Holland Publishing Company, 1977.

Mendelsohn, M. L., W. A. Kolman, B. Perry, and J. M. S. Prewitt: "Morphological Analysis of Cells and Chromosomes by Digital Computer." Sixth IBM Medical Symposium. 1964. New York.

Meyers, P. H., H. C. Becker, J. W. Sweeney, C. M. Nice, and W. J. Nettleson: "Evaluation of Computer-Retrieved Radiographic Image." *Radiology* 81: 201–6, 1963.

Michaels, A., B. Mittman, and C. R. Carlson: "A Comparison of the Relational and CODASYL Approaches to Data Base Management." *ACM Computing Surveys* 8(1):125–51, March 1976.

Mohr, J. R., E. R. Gabriele, V. Gaertner, B. Schwarz, K. D. Haehn, and P. L. Reichertz: "Purpose Means and Contents of Documentation in German General Practice." Medinfo 77 *Proceedings.* Amsterdam: North-Holland Publishing Company, 1977.

Mohr, J. R., D. D. Kaehn, and K. J. Dreibholz: "Analysis and Standardization of the Activities of the General Practitioner in Preparation for a Computer Oriented Information System." Medinfo 1974 *Proceedings.* Amsterdam: North-Holland Publishing Company, 1975.

Moore, R. T., M. C. Stark, and L. Cahn: "Digitizing Pictorial Information with a Precision Optical Scanner." Joint Annual Meeting of the American Society of Photogrammetry and the American Congress on Surveying and Mapping. 1964.

Murnaghan, J. H.: "Ambulatory Medical Care Data." *Med. Care,* 11(2) (Suppl.): 10–11, 1973.

National Center for Health Services Research and Development: *Comprehensive Hospital Computer Applications Program,* Vols. 1 and 2. 1972. National Technical Information Service, U.S. Department of Commerce, Springfield, Virginia.

National Library of Medicine: *Automation on Use of Computers in Laboratory Diagnosis – Recent Literature.* U. S. Department of Health, Education and Welfare, Periodical updating.

Norris, John A.: "Legal Aspects of Computer Use in Patient Interviewing and Screening." First National Conference on the Legal Aspects of Computer Use in Health Care Delivery. Boston, November 1974.

Norris, John A.: "Legal Aspects of Computer Use in Patient Therapy." First National Conference on the Legal Aspects of Computer Use in Health Care Delivery. Boston, November 1974.

Olsson, D. E.: "Automated Nurses' Notes – First Step in a Computerized Record System." *Hospitals, J.A.H.A.* 41:64, June 16, 1967.

Oppenheim, M., F. M. Delaney, M. Goldberg, W. Schumer, and A. G. Greenburg: "Simulation Model to Evaluate the Role of a Multiphasic Screening Unit in the Health Care Delivery System." Sixth Simulation Conference, p. 91. Tampa, Florida, March 1973.

Patrick, E. A.: "Pattern Recognition Applied to Surgery." *Computers in Biology and Medicine,* Vol. 4. New York: Pergamon Press, 1974.

Patrick, E. A.: "Review of Pattern Recognition in Medical Diagnosis and Consulting Relative to a New System Model." IEEE Systems, Man and Cybernetics Transactions, 1974.

Patrick, E. A.: "Expected Outcome Loss to Evaluate Medical Diagnosis and Treatments." *Proceedings,* 1976 Systems, Man, and Cybernetics Conference, of IEEE. Washington, D. C., November 1-3, 1976.

Patrick, E. A.: *Medical Decision Analysis Methodologies and Applications.* CRC Press, 1977. New York.

Patrick, E. A., et al.: "Compatible Medical Consulting and Diagnosis by Computer." Presented at the Second Illinois Conference on Medical Information Systems. Urbana, Illinois, September 24-25, 1975.

Peumans, W.: "Medical Computer Applications in Daily Practice by an Independent Group of Belgian Physicians." Medinfo 1974 *Proceedings.* Amsterdam: North-Holland Publishing Company, 1975.

Polli, G. J.: *Computers and Medicine, Special Report.* Chicago: American Medical Association, 1976.

Rawley, P. D.: "Quantitative Interpretation of Three-Dimensional Weakly Refractive Objects Using Holographic Interferometry." *J. Opt. Soc. Am.* 59: 1496-98, 1969.

Reichertz, P. L.: *Hospital Information Systems, Concept and Implementation of the Medical System Hannover (MSH),* pp. 153-86. Amsterdam: North-Holland Publishing Company, 1975.

Reichertz, P. L.: "Strategy Considerations for Hospital Information Systems," Medis '75 *Proceedings,* pp. 11-18. Tokyo, October 7-9, 1975.

Reichertz, P. L.: "Educational Requirements to Prepare for Expanded Usage of Information and Computer Science in Health." Computer Applications in Health Care Delivery, *7th Annual Meeting of the Society for Advanced Medical Systems,* pp. 113-20. Houston, New York, 1976.

Reichertz, P. L.: "Local and Regional Concept of Electronic Data Processing in West German Health Care Delivery." *The Computer in Health Care Systems in Some European Countries and in the United States* (ed. by E. Mase, M. L. Collen, and S. Gorini), pp. 99-124. Padua and London, 1976.

Riechertz, P. L.: "Realization of Data Protection by Software Techniques." IFIP WG 4.2: Working Conference on Realization of Data Protection in Health Information Systems. Kiel, June 23-25, 1976.

Rikli, A. E., and C. A. Caceres: "Computer Techniques for Electrocardiography. The Use of Computers by Physicians as a Diagnostic Aid." *Trans. N. Y. Acad. Sci.* 23:237-39, 1961.

Rodnick, J. E., and G. Widerhold: "A Review of Automated Ambulatory Medical Record Systems in the U. S." Medinfo 77 *Proceedings.* Amsterdam: North-Holland Publishing Company, 1977.

Rosenfield, V. L.: "A Chronological Team-Oriented Patient Record." *Hospital Administration in Canada,* pp. 36-40, June 1974.

Sauter, K., P. L. Reichertz, W. Weingartern, B. Schwarz, and D. Weigelt: " System-Controlled Structuring and Processing Tools for an Implemented Generalized Data Base Management System." *Angewandte Informatik* 8:348–49, 1976.

Schroer, B. J., and Herbert T. Smith: "Computers in Family Practice." *Proceedings*, p. 126. St. Louis, Missouri: MUMPS Users' Group, 1975.

Schwarz, Birgit, P. L. Reichertz, and J. R. Moehr: "An Analysis of Motivation Concerning EDP Implementation in General Practice." Medinfo 77 *Proceedings*. Amsterdam: North-Holland Publishing Company, 1977.

Shannon, R. H.: "Holy Family Hospital Medical Information System." *Problem-Directed and Medical Information Systems*, p. 175. New York: Intercontinental Medical Book Corporation, 1973.

Shannon, R. H.: "Networking Follow-Up." *Clinical Medicine and the Computer*, Minneapolis: SCM, 1974.

Shannon, R. H.: "The Second Wave, and Reexamination of Computers in Medicine." *Post Graduate Med.*, April 1975. (Reprinted by invitation in *Computer Med.*, September 1975.)

Sherman, H., and A. L. Kamaroff: "Ambulatory Care Project." Memeo, Cambridge, Massachusetts: Massachusetts Institute of Technology, Harvard Medical School, 1974.

Sherman, H., B. Reiffen, and A. L. Komaroff: "Aids to the Delivery of Ambulatory Medical Care." *IEEE Trans. Biomed. Eng.* 20(3):165–74, May 1973.

Shortliffe, E. H.: "Computer-Based Medical Consultation MYCIN." Elsevier Computer Science Library, p. 8. New York: Elsevier, 1976.

Slamecka, B.: "Objectives and Strategies for the Health Information Sciences." Medinfo 1974 *Proceedings*. Amsterdam: North-Holland Publishing Company, 1975.

Smith, A. L., Jr.: "Physician Data System." Paper given to Annual Meeting Society for Computer Medicine 1975. *Proceedings* Published by Coopers and Lybrand, 1975. New York.

Somers, J. B.: "A Computerized Nursing Care System." *Hospitals, J.A.H.A.* 45:93, April 16, 1971.

Sommerfelt, S. C.: "Conclusion on Medical Effectiveness and Consequences." *Proceedings,* Information Systems for Patient Care, 1975. Amsterdam: North-Holland Publishing Company, 1976.

Souder, D. E., et al.: "The Design of COSTAR V – A Generalizable Modular Medical Information System." Submitted for publication, *Proceedings of the 1976 MUMPS Users' Group Meeting.*

Spencer, W. A., and C. Vallbona: "Automated Data Processing of Medical Records." *J.A.M.A.* 191(11):121–23, 1965.

Spencer, W. A., and C. Vallbona: In *J.A.M.A.* 191(11):917–21, 1965.

Stallmann, R. W., and H. V. Pipberger: "Automatic Recognition of Electroncardiographic Waves by Digital Computer." *Circulat. Res.* 9:1138–43, 1961.

Sterling, T. D.: "Report on Progress in the Development of Visual Prostheses." *The New Outlook*, pp. 41–45, 1970.

Sterling, T. D., and S. V. Pollack: "Role of Statistics in the World of Computers." Reprint from *Ann. N. Y. Acad. Sci.*, 128 (Article 3):1108-15, 1966.

Sterling, T. D., and J. Weinkam: "A Versatile System for Three Dimensional Radiation Dose Computation and Diaplay, RTP." *Computer Programs in Bio Medicine* 2, pp. 178-92. Amsterdam: North-Holland Publishing Company, 1972.

Sterling, T. D., A. S. Glicksman, K. Knowlton, and J. Weinkam: "Three Dimensional Treatment Plan Display on Computer-Produced Films." Film Session, 12-14.

Sterling, T. D., and Harold Perry, and Jay Weinkam: "Automation of Radiation Treatment Planning VI — A General Field Equation to Calculate Percent Depth Dose in the Irradiated Volume of a Cobalt 60 Beam." *Br. J. Radiol.* 40:463-68, 1967.

Sterling, T. D., S. Pollack, and W. Spencer: "The Use of an Information System to Humanize Procedures in a Rehabilitation Hospital." *Int. J. Bio-Med. Computing*, pp. 51-57. London: Applied Science Publishers, Ltd. 1974.

Stimson, D. H., G. Charles, and C. L. Rogerson: "A Problem-Oriented Information System for a Primary Care Group Practice." Medinfo 77 *Proceedings*. Amsterdam: North-Holland Publishing Company, 1977.

Tarter, M. E. (with B. Hilberman, B. Kamm, and J. Osborn): "An Evaluation of Computer Based Patient Monitoring at Pacific Medical Center." *Computers Biomed. Res.* 8:447-460, 1975.

Temmerman, G. A. R.: "The Use of a Computer in General Practice: Basic Principles and Two Examples." Medinfo 1974 *Proceedings*. Amsterdam: North-Holland Publishing Company, 1975.

Teicholz, E.: LAB-LOG. Laboratory For Computer Graphics and Spatial Analysis, Harvard University, 1977 and 1978.

Tretiak, C. J., M. Eden, and W. Simon: In *Proceedings* 8th Int. Conf. on Med. Biol. Eng., Session 12-1. Chicago, 1969.

Tyler, C. R.: "Approaches to Hospital Information Systems." Medinfo 1974 *Proceedings*. Amsterdam: North-Holland Publishing Company, 1975.

Tzur, Baruch, S. Beilis, and E. Calabi: "Concepts of Data Structure for Clinical Laboratories Information System in Ambulatory Services." Medinfo 77 *Proceedings*. Amsterdam: North-Holland Publishing Company, 1977.

Vallbona, C., et al.: "A Computerized Patient Management System for a Community Clinic." Final Report. HSM 110-71-172, Department of Community Medicine, Baylor College of Medicine, Houston, Texas, 1975.

van Brunt, E. E., M. F. Collen, L. S. Davis, E. Besag, and S. J. Singer: "A Pilot Data System for a Medical Center." *Proc. IEEE* 57(11): 1969.

Wakefield, J. S., and S. R. Yarnall: *The History Database*, 3rd ed. Seattle, Washington: Medical Computer Services Association, 1975.

Warner, H. R., A. F. Toronto, and L. G. Veasy: "A Mathematical Approach to Medical Diagnosis. Application to Congenital Heart Disease." *J.A.M.A.* 177:177-83, 1961.

Waxman, B. D.: "COSTAR V – An Exportable Ambulatory Record and Management System." Sixth Annual Conference of the Society for Computer Medicine, Boston, November 12, 1976.

Wentz, H. S., H. L. Tindall, and N. J. Lenvanos: "Primary Care Research in a Model Family Practice Unit." *J. Fam. Pract.* 1:52–59, 1974.

Wied, G. L. (ed.): *Introduction to Quantitative Cytochemistry.* New York: Academic Press, 1966.

Wiederhold, G.: "Alternatives in Data Base Design for Ambulatory Records." *Proceedings,* Third Illinois Conference on Medical Information Systems. Department of Information Engineering, University of Illinois, Chicago, 1976.

Wilson, R. G.: "The Role of Computer/Communication Technology in Canadian Medicine." Medinfo 1977 *Proceedings.* Amsterdam: North-Holland Publishing Company, 1977.

Wolters, E., and P. L. Reichertz: "Problem Directed Interactive Transaction Management in Medical Systems." *Meth. Inform. Med.* 15:135–40, 1976.

Wood, E. H.: "Data Processing In Cardiovascular Physiology with Particular Reference to Roentgen Videodensitometry." *Proc. Staff Meetings Mayo Clin.* 39:849–65, 1964.

Yasnoff, W. A., and C. R. Carlson: "Relational Data Bases for Ambulatory Care." Medinfo 77 *Proceedings.* Amsterdam: North-Holland Publishing Company, 1977.

Yasnoff, W. A., and N. Justice: "COSTAR – Computer Stored Ambulatory Record." Information Flow Documentation, Laboratory of Computer Science, Massachusetts General Hospital, Boston, 1975.

Zimmerman, J.: *Dissemination of Computer Applications Via a Multi-Environment Scheme (MESCH).* BCL Monograph 248. St. Louis, Missouri: Biomedical Computer Laboratory, Washington University, 1974.

Zimmerman, J.: "Towards Generalized Automated Ambulatory Care Record Systems." Medinfo 77 *Proceedings.* Amsterdam: North-Holland Publishing Company, 1977.

Zimmerman, J., and D. Tao: "The MESCH (Multi-Environment Scheme) Approach to the Creation of Ambulatory-Care Record Systems." *Proceedings of the 1975 MUMPS Users' Group Meeting.* St. Louis, Missouri: MUMPS Users' Group, 1975.

Zimmerman, J., and C. R. Brigham: *MUMPS Application Design, Manuals for QUEST, a Simple Questionnaire Driver.* Monograph 300. St. Louis, Missouri: Biomedical Computer Laboratory, Washington University, 1976.

2
DESIGN PRINCIPLES OF COMPUTER—AIDED PHYSICIAN'S OFFICE SYSTEMS

Jan F. Brandejs, Ph.D.
Health Informatics Director
MDM Ltd., Toronto, Ontario, Canada

INTRODUCTION

Computers in the 1980s will play an increasing role in a busy physician's office, from taking over the chores of billing, accounting, and appointment scheduling to patient records, patient education, and follow-ups. The computer/communications technology is rapidly progressing from its infancy toward maturity. At this stage of development it will deliver the necessary information and free text processing power to physicians at costs they can afford to pay. In the past, for many reasons, but primarily because of prohibitive costs, doctors considered a switch from the present well-established manual procedures into computers as a premature or a very difficult change. Thus, until very recently computerization has had little impact on the ambulatory care environment despite some interesting projects in hospitals.[1]

During the past decade many attempts were made by computer manufacturers and systems and computer scientists, as well as a number of medical professionals, to implement computers in hospitals and physicians' offices. PROMIS (problem oriented medical information system),[2] COSTAR (computer stored ambulatory record system),[3] Technicon,[4] the Kaiser-Permanente system,[5] and the Mayo Clinic system, among others, contributed significantly to the emerging field of health informatics.[6] The 1980s should be more than just another decade because physicians, dentists, and other health care professionals have to choose between abandoning the previously designed systems and finding a new way of achieving systems that will serve them rather than the machine and computer vendors.

Explanations are manifold to justify the lack of interest displayed by physicians and their staff in computers. In my recent publication *Physician's Primer on Computers – Private Practice,*[7] I have stated that "computer-aided medical information systems are not so much technology as a well organized body of knowledge which will enable doctors to do things correctly." I am presenting the notion that the major challenge ahead is the mastering of new concepts and design principles of information systems acceptable to doctors and other health care professionals.

There is no doubt that the equipment (computers, VDTs, communication devices, mass storage, and such) is the basis of every computerized information system. There was, however, a narrow-minded concentration on the technology, and many proposals presented to physicians with regard to office computerization were overloaded with professional computer terminology. This was enough to discourage practicing physicians, their staff, and administrators of health care institutions from investigating closely the potentials of the computer/communications technology for the betterment of patient and office management.

Even if equipment and applications were made available to physicians at a reasonable cost, the new system must be accepted by both the physicians and their staff. The dissemination of relevant information in a well-organized publications must be considered one of the first tasks in the implementation of a medical information system. But there are problems. Physicians are not inclined to spend time on reading lengthy documents on computers, and are usually too busy or unable to attend formal training sessions in computer usage. The ancillary medical staff is so used to the present paper-based routines that they are unable to envisage the replacement of these procedures with a computerized system in which paper reports are considered the most unwanted product.

The past approach to the design of medical information systems was based on wrong assumptions regarding the attitudes of medical users. The major fallacy of the past systems was the concept of rigidly structured "menus" and printed reports. Such systems reenforced the traditional conservative thinking of physicians against computers. Moreover, programmers and project leaders of medical information systems were not concerned with the time and effort required by the medical professionals to use the system in their daily practice. As long as the computer-aided system is slower or is equal in performance to the present manual procedures, there is slim hope for computerized systems.

Until a few years ago, considerable confusion existed as to what may constitute an "acceptable" medical, clinical, and administrative system. Several vendors such as IBM, NCR, Honeywell, and Hewlett-Packard, among others, offer "medical/health care" application packages for their computers. In practice, however, the software covers mainly the billing and accounting procedures with very rudimentary linkage to patient scheduling, patient profiles, patient education, and so on. Presently very few vendors offer a comprehensive medical information system, the only exception being DEC (Digital Equipment Corporation). Based on the long development of COSTAR at the Laboratory of Medical

Computing, Massachusetts General Hospital, and at several dedicated implementation sites such as the Caledonian Medical-Surgical Clinic at Nanaimo, British Columbia, DEC is capable of offering a total clinical system for group practice. COSTAR system may be cost-justifiable in certain clinical environments.

In spite of the accomplishments of DEC the implementation of the new computerized technology in physicians' offices is still a risky endeavor for the medical profession as well as for the vendors. The risk level involved in setting up medical information systems is proportionally related to the attitudes of those involved. Such attitudes are shaped by tools and techniques within a dynamic environment. They are influenced, to a great degree, by skills and habits acquired through many years of traditional medical training. These deeply rooted traditions naturally create resentment toward every change. The implementation of computer/communications technology in the medical profession is a new venture and as such is easily subjected to abuse if safeguards are not wisely established.

MODULAR APPROACH

A modular medical information system is a package or set of mutually interrelated application programs working as a whole for a purpose specified by the users. The structure of data files and the flexibility of the system's software (e.g., operating system − OS) may determine how effectively the applications work together in order to minimize the input of medical data and to maximize the satisfaction of the users with regard to the output. The needs of medical users may vary widely, depending on the type of practice and its location. Flexibility and ability to customize or tailor the programs to the specific requirements of each practice must be the prime consideration of the modular concept.

In a busy practice, physicians have little time to think about the new forms of office and patient management. In a free market (fee-for-service) patient care environment it is still difficult to establish clearly what kind of procedures may improve the present system. No two doctors have the same education or experience in providing services for their patients; nor will they agree on what constitute, for instance, good patient records. The same disease process does not present itself the same way twice in two different patients. Therefore, there will be numerous perceptions of the role of computers and their utilization for medical practice. Some physicians will gain rapid understanding of and skill in computer use in limited applications (e.g., billing). On the other hand, the establishment of well and cost-efficient "complete" systems, covering a wide variety of applications, is a very slow, time-consuming learning process. Furthermore, if an attempt is made to deliver and install a medical system "overnight" (a "turnkey" system), the resulting frustrations may prevent the physician and his/her ancillary staff from further improving their skills because there has been no adjustment to change. The modular approach assumes a natural growth, as in the development of body from fetus to adult.

The introduction of computerization in private practice is a human-dependent process. It is a continuing development entailing many changes in human behavior over a long time. However, such a fundamental process of change must be based on the modular approach, from simple or most needed applications such as patient registration and billing toward the more sophisticated and more time-consuming, such as patient records. The clinic managers, or in some cases the vendors or consultants, may play an important role in the modular system. They have to identify the interrelationships, sequence, and priorities of each application and module relevant to the needs of the particular practice. They also must assess the major factors at play during the transition period from manual methods to the computer-aided system. As manual operations such as filing and jobs with repetitive and mechanical assignments become redundant, one of the major issues that confronts each practice is the fear that clinic staff will be replaced by the computer. Usually, however, staff reduction is accomplished through normal attrition and retraining for other jobs associated with computer operations.

The system architects should be able to explain and demonstrate that the computer should never interfere in the physician/patient relationship. Patients expect that the physician will render compassionate medical care. Since privacy and confidentiality are prime concerns to the physician and the patient, both may view an ostentatiously displayed terminal or noisy printer with suspicion. The computer operation should become a natural part of investigation and treatment procedures. An open-minded cooperation, a regular exchange of timely information, and a tolerance of anxieties, fears, and expectations among the physician, the patient, and the vendor will mold a team of knowledgeable people dedicated to the implementation and usage of user-oriented systems in the ambulatory care setting and clinical investigations.

Every vendor, consultant, or systems engineer will argue that his/her system is user-oriented. To prove this assertion, it is necessary to examine the operation of the computerized system under the constraints that apply to a busy medical office. For example, is it possible to make an appointment for a patient while he/she is waiting in the office and at the same time be in touch with a patient who is calling by phone? Or does it take minutes to select the appointment application from the general menu? If the latter is true, the system is not user-oriented because the programmer developed programs not suitable for use in an ambulatory care environment. In other words, a receptionist who is comfortable when sitting at the terminal with access to the stored information on free appointment slots, doctors, and/or laboratory and radiology scheduling, feels confident and competent when dealing with patients.

It should be pointed out that the use of a system in the medical practice does not require an on-line, real-time access to all stored information by all staff at any given time. This may have been a condition for the operation of systems in hospitals. Practicing physicians can treat their patients, in emergency situations or in case of computer shutdown, without any information. In such events the updating of the files can be made later. In the case of computer malfunction, for example, the receptionist can make the appointments for the patients on a preliminary basis, update the files as soon as the computer is functioning again, and inform the patients by telephone of any changes. The same premise is valid in case of the malfunctioning of computerized patient records, billing, or accounting.

The concept of a viable and cost-efficient system is based, in the first place, on the acceptance of the system by physicians and their staff through gradual implementation of logically interconnected applications. The accompanying figure portrays the concept of a system that presently is being tested in Canada. It is based on the logical premise that the hub of each physician's office is patient records. The system under investigation consists of three basic applications: (1) appointments (time management module); (2) billing and accounting (financial module); and (3) cumulative patient profiles (medical record module). These three applications are referred to as the A-B-C of medical information systems.

Time Management Module

In present procedures patient scheduling, appointments, and management of doctors' time, are usually considered as applications having a relatively low priority. However, up to 80 percent of billing data is generated by the appointment and patient registration application. The computerization of patient scheduling solves the "nightmare" of medical practice — that is, when the patient or the doctor does not appear as scheduled. The rescheduling of the patient is an easy task for a computerized system, whereas it is a nearly impossible assignment within a manual booking system. The analogy with airline scheduling is the best example of the necessity for computerized patient booking. Needless to say, no airline could exist today without a computer.

Few doctors are able to deliver maximum effort for more than four to five hours without a break. Short breaks are important factors in achieving optimal productivity without an increased rate of errors. Long hours in the office and even working through the lunch hour are usually dictated by disorganized scheduling of patients. The major problem associated with a smooth flow of patients is in the proper time allocation or the uncertainty of how much time is required for each visit. In addition, often the physician is late, or an emergency situation has occurred, or the patient is late, did not show up, or has just walked in.

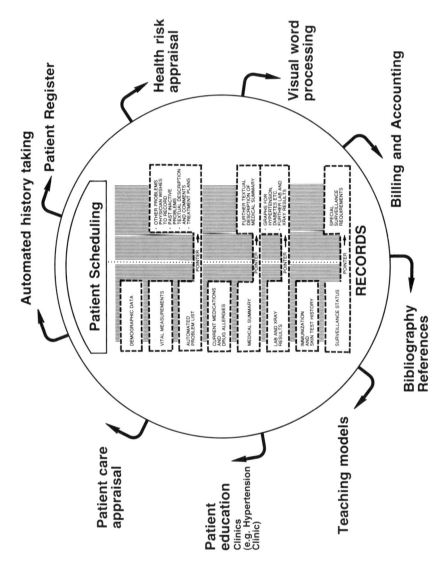

Figure 1. Design principles of computer-aided physician's office system.

In order to cope with all these unpredictable factors encountered in a busy practice, the most effective technique is scheduling patients in waves. The wave approach, which schedules patients with similar problems in clusters rather than at regular intervals, is the key factor in using flexible but planned scheduling in an individually tailored patient work load. As a first step for the physician, a timetable must be created to show his regular or basic schedule for days with the average number of patients, an expanded schedule allowing for same-day "drop-ins" and "call-ins," and an epidemic schedule for unusual situations. If the doctor works different hours on different days, more than one schedule must be established and stored in the computer memory. Each schedule specifies in detail, hour by hour, the number of appointment slots. The type of appointment, such as "regular," "demand" (drop-ins or same-day call-ins), and "epidemic" (to be used only in extreme circumstances), should be indicated. The regular appointments could be further categorized as, for example, check-ups, hospitals, institutions, nursing homes, and so on. The purpose of the program is to store a set of timetables for the physician whether he/she is in solo, partnership, or group practice.

Financial Module

This module uses data captured by the registration and patient scheduling procedures. The quality of medical services rendered, of the organizational level of appointments, and of medical records has a great influence on the quality of billing. If patient scheduling and medical recording are disorganized, the inadequacy of these operations is then directly projected into messy and costly patient billing. The purpose of the computerized billing is to provide the physician with an easy yet flexible method of preparing information on charges and billing documents for direct patient or third-party billing. Commercially available billing (accounts receivable) and accounting packages are recommended for modification. A unified chart of accounts is promoted as a means for better statistical and financial analyses on a national level.

Medical Records Module

As the medical records module is the most sophisticated among all applications, it necessitated the development of new record-oriented languages, such as MUMPS (Massachusetts General Hospital Utility Multi-programming System)[8] and MUG (Medical University Generator).[9] Direct inquiries are made through video terminals in the care areas. The printed medical records or patient summaries are available on demand to physicians for each scheduled visit. Computer-aided records, their purpose, substance, style, format, and content, could, for many years to come, be a major source of controversy in the use of the module of medical information systems for ambulatory care.

For a better understanding of the complex and sometimes emotionally charged medical recording issue, the purpose of patient records may be summarized as follows. They serve as an aide-memoire to the doctor as to what happened to his patient prior to the present appointment. They are also used in the following ways: as a cumulative aide-memoire over a range of patients (e.g., a family), if such information is required for the specific specialty; as guides to investigation and treatment (i.e., complete history, physical examinations, multiphasing screening, laboratory and X-ray reports, and such); as monitoring and predicting tools of the progress of the patient's illness by using logically structured patient progress notes; as stimuli for developing new ideas about the diagnoses and treatment of patients by deploying the concept of feedback (in hypertension and diabetes clinics) and other computer-based innovations; as tools for analyzing data as they arise in the medical record; as a means of searching for correlations of symptomatic and therapeutic patterns; and as an aid for medical audit and peer review.

The major blocks of information included in the computerized medical records are as follows: demographic data, which include emergency information and a list of hospitalizations; vital signs and measurements; complete as well as temporary problem list; current medications and drug allergies; patient history and list of patient problems; laboratory and radiological reports; immunization and skin tests; patient follow-up; billing status; and, if required, risk factor assessment. Substantial modifications of this concept are expected as soon as more practicing physicians become involved in this field.

Design Principles

In summary, the modular system design should be based on the following principles:

1. The system should be built in a modular fashion rather than in a random, haphazard way.

2. The cost for the use of the A-B-C modules, including word processing, should not exceed the cost of the present manual system or a maximum of $400.00 per month per physician.

3. The response time to any on-line inquiry should be less than three seconds.

4. The inquiry terminals (video display units) should be compact enough to fit into any examination room.

5. The programming language used must be flexible and thus enable the programmer to orient the system toward the user.

6. The computer should require minimal technical arrangements such as adequate air conditioning and power supply.

7. The system must be operated by people with minimal training, usually by the staff.

8. The funding of the development and the requisition of the equipment must be based on sound investment arrangements, reflecting the present high interest rates.

9. The maintenance of the computer/communications technology must be readily available, preferably from one source.

10. Privacy and confidentiality of the stored data must be ensured with the physician as an ultimate guarantor.

Conclusion

The basic modules of the medical information system should cover the major needs of practicing physicians and, in group practice, the needs of the clinic management. The implementation process of the first level consists of the following major activities: computer testing, staff training, equipment installation, system conversion, new systems operation testing period, and comparison of planned vs. actual results.

The testing of the new system should be done, if possible, outside the practice. Hardware is tested for reliability of disk drives, quality of printing, and the noise levels of the printer and disk units. The selected applications should be tested to determine how specific requirements of the medical practice are being met. Staff training is one of the most important activities during all phases of system implementation. As soon as firm contractual arrangements are satisfactorily concluded, the medical staff should be exposed to several levels of indoctrination. Installation of the computer, terminals, other hardware, and equipment is usually left to the vendor's experts. System conversion is a serious affair with little or no fun in it. Patient registration files, physicians' appointment schedules, and lists of most frequently used diagnostic codes should be entered into the computer memory and tested for completeness and accuracy. Incomplete files must be flagged for completion during the next patient visit. All manual files should be maintained for a reasonable time as a system back-up. Vendors' experts should be involved in the conversion process as much as possible. After several months of operation, assessment of results should be undertaken by senior staff or senior partners. The vendor representative should also be present for his advice on the minor changes that may be required.

REFERENCES

1. Collen, M. F. (ed.): *Hospital Computer Systems.* New York: Wiley, 1974.
2. Hurst, J. W., and H. K. Walker (eds.): *The Problem-oriented System.* New York: Medcom, 1972.
3. Barnett, G. O.: *Computer-stored Ambulatory Records.* Boston: Laboratory of Computer Science, Massachusetts General Hospital, 1977.
4. Watson, R. J.: "A Large-scale Professionally Oriented Medical Information System — Five Years Later." *J. Med. Computing 1* (2): 1978.
5. Davis, L. S., and T. A. Simacek: "Distributed Data Base Medical Informations Systems." *Proceedings*, Information Systems for Patient Care. Amsterdam: North-Holland, 1976.
6. Brandejs, J. F.: *Health Informatics.* Amsterdam: North-Holland, 1976.
7. Brandejs, J. F., and C. G. Pace: *Physician's Primer on Computers — Private Practice.* Lexington, Massachusetts: Lexington Books, 1979.
8. Barnett, G. O., et al: "MUMPS: A Support for Medical Information Systems." *Med. Informatics 1:* 1976.
9. GEAC Canada Ltd. *GEAC 8000 System Description.* Markham, 1979.

3
CRITERIA FOR SELECTION OF A FEASIBLE MEDICAL OFFICE COMPUTER SYSTEM

Peter V. Weston, San Antonio, Texas

DEVELOPING AN EXPERTISE

Computer science has its own language and buzz words. This language must be understood if users wish to communicate with personnel from the industry. Once industry jargon is understood, the computer no longer appears as a mysterious black box that can perform supernatural or magic tricks.

The initial knowledge can be gained either by attending a course on "Introduction to Computers," offered by the continuing education departments of most universities or community colleges, or by obtaining appropriate materials from the many "computer stores" that are proliferating throughout the country as a direct result of the availability of home computers.

Several general-interest magazines are now available that publish instructive articles on computer basics as well as more advanced articles.

The application of computers to medical practice is receiving the attention of more and more professionals. "Electronic Data Processing for a Medical Office" is a course offered by Practice Productivity Incorporated, a medical management consulting firm in Atlanta, Georgia. This course is designed to acquaint physicians and their office personnel with the state of the art and to provide assistance in selection criteria. Courses sponsored by specific manufacturers or vendors could be biased.

As part of his education, the physician could consider buying a small home computer such as a TRS 80, Apple II, PET, etc. He would thereby have a machine to use at his convenience to develop some computer skills. This suggestion is not meant to recommend that each physician redevelop the wheel by writing all his own programs but rather that each physician develop skills so that he can better use the wheel.

Home computer systems can be developed to support a small limited practice. However, as the practice grows and new applications are developed, a larger system, such as a mini or micro, will have to be acquired. When this happens, and after the appropriate tax deductions have been taken, the computer can be given to the physician's children, or it can be put to additional stand-alone uses such as patient education programs or taking patient histories.

Several physician-oriented periodicals such as *Physicians Microcomputer Report*[1] and *Computers in Medicine*[2] are available. These publications are very informative but require at least an elementary understanding of computers.

The American Society of Internal Medicine recently developed a guide designed to serve as an educational process for internists and their office staffs and to help them determine whether or not a computer would work well in their individual practices.[3] In addition, this guide offers advice to buyers and lists questions to ask prospective vendors.

Buying a computer can be likened to acquiring an automobile. The purchaser has to have a basic knowledge of the applications so that the decision can be made as to whether to acquire a dune buggy, sports car, family car, jeep, pickup, or tractor. A further analogy is the similarity between computer salesmen and used car salesmen. This is especially true of those representatives with sales backgrounds. Agents who have technical electronic data processing experience are better able to offer expert advice.

Nevertheless, the more knowledgeable and the more involved the physician, the less the likelihood of being hoodwinked!

EVALUATING NEEDS

A computer system must produce significant benefits in business efficiency and productivity to justify the cost and time expenditure. As every practice is unique, each physician or group of physicians must thoroughly review each aspect of their practice that is amenable to automation, evaluate the computer marketplace, and perform a cost/benefit study.

Perhaps the greatest benefit of such a review will be a personal understanding of the intricacies of the existing system, which can help in analyzing requirements and expectations from a computer.

The cost of processing charges, receipts, and generation of statements is usually readily calculable from the salaries of personnel. However, this figure must be modified by factoring in intangibles such as punctuality of statement mailing, quality and appearance of the statements, and the number of phone calls verifying statement figures. The evaluation should also review the entire collection process, including confirmation of address and telephone numbers at each office visit, objective analysis of insurance filing procedures, practice statistics, and internal controls that discourage mishandling of funds.

The next step is the documentation of the number of transactions performed in the present system. The physician must know the number of daily transactions (charges, receipts, new and established patients) and the number of monthly tasks (statements, collection notices, and insurance claim forms). In addition, a decision has to be made regarding the number of patients about whom historical accounting data are to be retained.

Once this review is completed, the size of the proposed system can be determined. The amount of memory and the amount of disc storage needed are directly proportional to the number of patients to be kept on the Master File, the number of transactions to be stored, and the time frame over which immediate access to data is to be available.

Applications other than accounts receivable management will predicate additional storage requirements.

Other areas in which electronic data processing can be applied include:

Accounts receivable management
Statistical reporting
Productivity profiles on each physician
Business accounting
    Payroll
    Accounts payable
    General ledger
Appointment scheduling
Word processing
    Referral letters
    Medical records
    Histories and physicals
    Operative and consultation reports

Each computerized task must be assigned an anticipated benefit, which can be:

1. Payroll saving by reduction in personnel
2. Increased cash flow
3. Improved collection techniques
4. Improved financial reporting
5. Improved efficiency
6. Improved productivity
7. Improved medical records
8. Improved and more efficient reporting of medical findings to referring physicians, etc.

It must be emphasized that a computer cannot organize a disorganized practice. If this is the situation, the weaknesses must be diagnosed and treatment initiated before computerization is considered.

DEFINING REQUIREMENTS

We now have reached the point at which needs can be accurately defined, and these needs must be communicated to vendors so that the physician can search for an appropriate system instead of altering requirements to suit a generalized system that vendors might have available. By providing vendors with specific requirements, the physician is buying a system and is not being *sold* a prepackaged configuration that might not be relevant to the practice.

The document asking for bids is referred to as a "Request for Proposal" (RFP). This RFP must be comprehensive and explicit. The RFP should be divided into categories, and in the covering letter sent with each request, vendors should be asked to adopt the same clear divisions in their responses. In addition, the letter should contain a closure date and should inform the vendors that their proposal will become part of any negotiated contract.

The following guide is based on the outline recommended by Naus.[4]

1. Description of Present System

This is an attempt to convey to the potential vendors as much information as possible regarding the nature and scope of the present system. It should include the bookkeeping method used, the personnel in the business office, and the equipment.

It should also tabulate:

1. Number of new patients per month
2. Number of transactions per month
3. Number of statements per month
4. Number of insurance claims per month
5. Number of patients with active accounts (patients with outstanding balances)
6. Total number of patients to be kept on line at any time

2. Five-Year Operating Plan

This is included to ensure that the proposed system is expandable to accommodate the proposed growth and expansion without significant alteration of the basic configuration.

3. Application Specifications

The vendors are asked to describe in detail the proposed system. The following is an excerpt from a RFP written by the author:

Please follow each question with as brief a response as is possible. If reference material is necessary, please supply it. Reference the material in your answer by including the title of the document, page(s) and paragraph(s). Please do not answer a question simply by providing a reference manual.

List all changes or upgrades in equipment and associated costs based on our five year plan. Include any software modifications as part of that upgrade. Please list all operating characteristics of proposed equipment.

Provide a functional description of the proposed system. Describe operational procedures, special features, error handling capabilities, data recovery, throughput and response times.

Provide examples of all report and CRT display formats. If examples are not available, describe the input and output concepts of the proposed system.

Describe the form and content of the documentation to be provided.

It is not the purpose of this chapter to define the software requirements of an ideal medical office system, but it is the responsibility of the writer of the RFP to break down each application program into subunits and specifics. For example, if it is important to continue with five-digit alphameric account codes rather than seven-digit alphabetic codes used in the IBM 5110, this must be so specified.

Other similar specifics could include:

1. Checks for missing patient tickets
2. Accounts receivable aging on demand or by other criteria, such as over 90 days with balance over $200
3. Home as well as business telephone numbers
4. Purging capability
5. Etc., etc.

4. Hardware Configuration

For each component, one should ask for the purchase price, lease, and monthly maintenance charge.

Supplemental hardware information should answer questions concerning:

1. Floor space required.
2. Type of flooring.

3. Electrical requirements.
4. Air-conditioning requirements.
5. The maximum number of input devices with the proposed configuration. With upgrades. Whether modems can be used and how many.
6. The type of CPU memory.
7. How much memory is available.
8. As video display terminals are added, whether core requirements will increase.
9. The maximum mass storage.
10. What types of mass storage units are available.
11. What the disc drive capacity is.
12. Whether discs are fixed, removable, or both.
13. How much time is necessary to copy a disc.
14. If several video display units are operating at the same time, whether each can be processing a different task.
15. How many characters can be displayed at one time, and on how many lines.
16. How far from the CPU video display units can be located without tele-communications.
17. Whether terminals can be utilized on-line from remote offices.
18. How many different types of printing devices can be incorporated into the system, and at what speeds they operate.
19. Whether printers can be swapped.
20. Whether all components are manufactured and supported by the vendors.
21. If a change of printers is required, what the cost will be.

5. Hardware Maintenance

The following questions should be asked:

1. What is the specific time period covered under the maintenance agreement?
2. Can additional coverage be added? By unit?
3. Are all maintenance costs, including transportation, parts, labor, and equipment, included? If no, please explain.
4. What is the normal preventive maintenance schedule for this configuration?
5. What is the expected delay time for on-call personnel to arrive at the installation?
6. What is the down-time experience with the proposed equipment? By unit?
7. What is considered excessive down time?
8. How many customer engineers are located at your nearest office?

9. How many are actually trained on all units included in your proposed system?
10. What are your rates for service other than on scheduled coverage? Parts? Etc.?
11. Do you keep spare parts at your support location?
12. Do you have a system comparable to the proposed configuration at your support location?

6. Back-up Installations

These questions should be included:

1. Where is the nearest location of a compatible back-up system that could be used in the event of excessive down time?
2. Who is responsible for making provisions for this back-up?
3. Do you have a compatible system in your office?
4. Are there any established user groups in a relatively close location?
5. Include a list of compatible systems within a 100-mile radius.

7. Software Definition

As software is the heart of the system, the RFP must demand a detailed listing of all the systems and application software together with a brief narrative outline. The cost of each program and the estimated cost of modification should also be requested.

Supplemental software information could include the following:

(a) Programming languages
1. The languages supported by the system
2. The language in which the software applications are written
3. The cost of additional compilers
4. The cost of a word-processing package
(b) Personnel — The availability in the local area of industry-trained persons
(c) Miscellaneous — Answers to these questions:
1. Is all application software to be written, program packages, or both?
2. Will vendor agree in a contract to complete modifications as required?
3. Will vendor warrant the application software as specified?
4. Can the actual programs being utilized at another user location be seen?

5. Prior to equipment delivery, will the conversion of patient files, etc., to the system be scheduled and completed?
6. Is the documentation fully provided in an understandable form?
7. Are all costs quoted in one sum or separately?

8. Installation Schedule

The vendor should be asked to provide a step-by-step schedule of:

1. The proposed delivery date for hardware
2. A list of all pre-installation tasks and associated responsibilities with suggested completion dates in detail
3. A periodic review method to ensure completion of those required tasks
4. List of applications implementation schedules by priority applications
5. Post-installation requirements and support
6. Guidance with reference to forms design and necessary supplies
7. The parallel-run time frame

9. Education

The vendor must be asked to specify the amount of training to be given to the office personnel *and the physicians,* and the location, dates, and cost of education courses.

Requests for Proposals should be sent to as many vendors as possible, because the more proposals submitted, the greater the choice and the greater the likelihood of achieving the ideal system.

A vendor who is not prepared to produce a proposal that can be easily scrutinized probably does not have a suitable system, or is unwilling to spend the necessary time to design one. In the latter case, it is better to discover this reluctance before making the investment of time and money.

FEASIBILITY STUDY

In all likelihood, the range of costs of the systems offered in the submitted proposals will vary enormously, with some probably twice as much as others. Nevertheless, a cost/benefit analysis can now be performed.

While this is not a complex task, an accountant should be involved because the cost of the equipment (hardware, software, and installation costs) should be spread over a five-year period and the appropriate tax credits and depreciations factored in. The final figures should be compared with the costs of the current system modified by the dollar figures that were arbitrarily given to the improved efficiency and production that automation can provide.

It is possible that the feasibility study will show that the time is not right for automation of the practice. Nevertheless, the exercise will not have been in vain, as a considerable amount of expertise will have been gleaned, and subsequent reading may well reveal new systems that will be cost-effective as further applications of software for microcomputers are generated.

VENDOR SELECTION

By this time, the physician or physicians should have made one of four choices:

1. To continue with the present system.
2. To use a service bureau with either batch processing or a data entry device with real-time inquiry capability.
3. To purchase a turnkey system — that is, a hardware and software package that is complete so that the user can operate it without having to write or obtain additional software support.
4. To purchase the hardware and independently develop customized software. Custom programming allows the user to design the system while maintaining flexibility for upgrading and enhancements. Cost overruns can be very high, debugging problems are frequent, and implementation delays are common. Past performance history should be a key consideration for this choice.

Because very few hardware manufacturers have the full software that is needed, the physician (or purchaser) will have to review the reputation of the manufacturer and the software vendor, topics that will be discussed in detail in the following pages.

MANUFACTURER

Reputation

The reputations of the major manufacturers need not be belabored; but only the top five or six companies can be considered absolutely secure, and numerous smaller companies have collapsed or are diverting their energies to other endeavors. In addition, we are now seeing numerous (and often short-lived) OEMs (outside equipment manufacturers) who have sprung up in the marketplace. These are companies that purchase components from various sources and box them under their own name. Should a company fail, long-term support of the equipment must be considered suspect, and interfacing problems associated with replacing components could be very expensive. Length of time in business, financial history, availability of service, and down-time response must be thoroughly evaluated.

Hardware Expansion Capability

When the user growth rate has exceeded the limitations of the system, or the potential reality of such a situation becomes imminent, system expandability becomes paramount. At this time, the existing system has to be disposed of, and the next larger system purchased. If this is the case, many manufacturers will not offer to trade in or "buy back" the equipment on hand to help ease the transition. If a nonexpandable system is considered, these policies should be investigated before signing a contract.

On the other hand, some systems on the market are modularly expandable. When the system limits are reached, additional components or peripherals can be added that will increase the system capacity (i.e., memory add-on, additional disc or tape units for external storage, new terminals for data entry or inquiry, additional second printer, etc.). If the potential user foresees future growth, these considerations should be studied.

System Software Support

System software is software supplied by the hardware manufacturer to ease the burden of application software development — especially the more common but complex functions such as sort/merge, random access, date conversion, screen formatting, data entry, data compaction or compression, etc. The lack of such software support can add many months of development effort and increase costs considerably, especially if the user is anticipating software development.

Availability of Maintenance and Down-Time Response

The availability of service and the proximity of the service organization are obviously vital factors to consider. The average response time for service calls must be investigated — no one wants to be held up for several hours or days awaiting maintenance personnel. The number of personnel locally, availability of spare parts locally, and availability of back-up systems locally are key factors to consider. The willingness of a manufacturer to provide substitute equipment, should the system require extensive maintenance, is a positive factor.

Software Compatibility in Upgrades

Should you decide to purchase a system in an "expandable family" of computers, ensure that the software will be compatible with each expansive step. Software conversion costs in an upgrade should be considered prior to purchase.

SOFTWARE SELECTION MAINTENANCE

Ascertain that the software vendor thoroughly understands the identified needs, both current and future, as evidenced by the completeness of the proposal. The integrity, reputation, business record, and financial stability of the software supplier should be evaluated as closely as that of the hardware manufacturer.

The answers to the following questions will assist greatly in the final decision:

1. How long have the suppliers been offering the services?
2. Have they provided a copy of their financial report for the last three years?
3. How far away are they located?
4. How many medical offices do they service?
5. Have they kept up with changes in the field?
6. How good is their "service"?
7. How do other doctors feel about that service?
8. Who does the work of conversion?
9. Do they have back-up equipment?
10. Will they train office personnel?
11. Will they assist with systems work and forms design?
12. What happens when service is discontinued?

SELECTION CRITERIA

From the proposals, a short list of three to five suppliers should be made and these vendors interviewed. Permission should be obtained to visit existing installations to see the system *in action.* During these visits, ask in-depth questions, including those of staff acceptability and ease in training new personnel. A key question in assessing the equipment is to ask the users what, if any, improvements they would recommend.

If one physician is primarily responsible for the final recommendations, it is wise to document the reasons for recommendations (see accompanying evaluation form). This process can be simplified to the selection of the lowest-cost vendor if all significant factors (tangible and intangible) are priced and added to, or subtracted from, the total "system life" cost as presented by the vendor.

Now an objective evaluation can be performed and a decision made. The decision is documented and can be understood by all.

CONTRACTS

Once the final selection is made, a contract must be negotiated. This is an extremely valuable document that will specifically spell out the guarantees and re-

Five-Year Cost	Vendor A	Vendor B	Vendor C
Hardware	$	$	$
Maintenance	$	$	$
Software	$	$	$
Training	$	$	$
Supplies	$	$	$
Utilities	$	$	$
Staff	$	$	$
Intangible Benefits			
Better maintenance service	$	$	$
More up-to-date hardware	$	$	$
Extra programming language	$	$	$
Quicker delivery	$	$	$
Better proposal	$	$	$
Local company	$_____	$_____	$_____
Relative cost	$_____	$_____	$_____

sponsibilities of each party. It is therefore imperative to commission a lawyer experienced in drawing up contracts.

This document must:

1. Specifically define all guarantees and services.
2. Describe how potential difficulties and areas of conflict will be resolved.
3. Provide written documentation explaining the agreement-commitment between the parties.
4. Provide recourse and remedies for both parties. (For example, if the vendor goes out of business, all source programs should be available, in escrow if necessary.)
5. Contain hardware and software specifications, including the listing of *all* software programs.
6. Provide details of maintenance contracts.
7. Confirm compatibility of components and ability to expand upward.
8. Incorporate the claims made by the vendors in their response to the original RFP.
9. Cover payment terms.
10. Define installation schedule.
11. Detail specifics of training to physicians and personnel.
12. Give warranties of ownership of equipment and the right to continue using the software.

Depending on the circumstances and recommendations by the attorney, additional clauses can be added.

EPILOGUE

Notwithstanding everything that has been written, one should not, at the first attempt, buy a comprehensive system. Rather, start off with a system with a limited number of applications, and grow with the system.

SUMMARY

The purchase of a computer must be considered a major undertaking, and must be divided into several distinct steps.

1. Developing an Education. To make intelligent decisions, the physician must have a general knowledge of computer principles and terminologies to enable him to communicate with the industry.

2. Defining the Practice Needs. The billing and accounting procedures must be analyzed in depth and the study documented. At this point, the practice needs can be specifically written out.

3. Writing a Request for Proposal. This is a standard procurement device and is a comprehensive statement to interested vendors asking for a proposal that will satisfy the defined needs.

4. Feasibility Study. This is a cost/benefit study to evaluate the justification of electronic data processing.

5. Vendor Selection. Once the decision has been made to purchase a computer, the respondents to the RFP must be critically evaluated, and not only by the ability to provide the system requested; also each company must be scrutinized and existing systems inspected.

By documenting the real costs and the intangible benefits, the company with the most cost-effective system can be chosen.

6. Contract Negotiations. The final and most important negotiations are reserved for the contract(s). The services of an attorney skilled in contracts are mandatory.

REFERENCES

1. *Physicians Microcomputer Report,* Editor, Dr. Gerald M. Orosz, P.O. Box 6483, Lawrenceville, New Jersey 08648.

2. *Computers and Medicine,* American Medical Association, 535 North Dearborn Street, Chicago, Illinois 60610. A practical guide to computers in practice.

3. *The Internist,* The American Society of Internal Medicine, December 1978–January 1979.

4. Naus, F., Practice Productivity, Inc., 2000 Clearview Avenue, Atlanta, Georgia.

4
"PRAKTICE"—AN ADVANCED CLINICAL INFORMATION SYSTEM

E.R. Gabrieli, M.D., Buffalo, New York

INFORMATION DEFICIT IN CLINICAL MEDICINE

Medical knowledge, as it is organized into medical textbooks, is essentially the formalized corpus of past clinical experience. The two-volume textbook of pathology by Anderson[1] is 2,148 pages long, and the *Textbook of Medicine* by Beeson and McDermott[2] is 1,892 pages long. A full set of textbooks of basic sciences and clinical specialties would comprise about 60,000 pages, representing the current corpus of medical knowledge. This awesome quantity of knowledge represents about ten times the capacity of the human memory. Further, today, these textbooks, in some areas, are already obsolete when printed, owing to the current pace of progress in medicine.

This vast volume of medical information, no longer memorizable, has created a major problem in clinical medicine. Our medical leaders recognize that our patients no longer receive the "best" diagnosis/therapy. There is an ill-defined gap between existing knowledge and actual clinical care. This growing gap is the *information deficit*, the concern of our decade.

The rate of growth of medical knowledge can be determined by studying the evolution of our current knowledge during the last 50–60 years.[3] According to our studies, during the last 50 years the average annual growth rate of clinical medicine has been 5 percent, compounded annually.

Growth of medical knowledge was still manageable in the 1930s, but not in the 1940s. Medicine had to accept the concept of specialization. This measure reduced the expected scope of expertise and increased the length of training. For at least two decades specialization was effective in controlling the knowledge deficit, but in the late 1960s the proliferation of such specialties reflected the same problem. Today, there are more than 100 recognized specialties, an indication of our difficulty in learning what should be known.

In the United States, the problem of the 1970s was to cope with the growing knowledge deficit. Mandatory continuing education of the practitioner, reexamination, relicensing, and various peer review programs are some of the symptoms. It is quite apparent that our traditional method of learning and recall is undergoing great difficulties. The purpose of this chapter is to describe a man–machine system where "computable" knowledge (i.e., computerized information) assists the failing memory of the physician, to help in decision functions.

INFORMATION COMPONENTS OF CLINICAL DECISIONS

In his clinical work, the physician uses several different types of information. For the sake of this discussion, we may categorize them as follows:

1. *Patient-related information:* Current complaints, recent clinical course, past medical history, and genetic and social background.
2. *Related clinical experiences:* Experience with similar cases.
3. *Related formal medical knowledge:* Segments of textbooks pertinent to diagnosis, therapy, prognosis, and clinical course.
4. *Theories, concepts, experimental hypotheses:* Proposals by researchers working in related areas, to explain the underlying pathophysiology, or to describe new methods of therapy.

Possessing these four types of pertinent data, the physician could make scientific and rational decisions in the form of diagnosis, therapy, and prognosis.

Considering these four categories of information used in clinical medicine, we can define the scope of computable information as *pertinent information affecting the clinical decision.* We propose that the technology should provide the computable information, in order to assist the physician in his information-dependent decisions. Such a computer support of medicine should be in real time, interactive, simple to use, comprehensive, and practical. The purpose here is to briefly describe our approach to such a medical information system, which has as its goal to provide the pertinent facts to the physician so that information-dependent clinical decisions can be limited only by the existing frontlines of knowledge, not by the limited capacity of the human memory.

THE MAN-MACHINE SYSTEM

In our own thinking process, we handle *ideas.* These ideas are the building blocks of our cognitive mental process. When we wish to share our ideas with others, we *verbalize* them. This transformation of our ideas into natural language words and sentences is the first step in medical communication. The success of this communication depends mainly upon (1) the fidelity of the verbalization of our ideas and (2) the ability of the receiver of our communication to fully comprehend the intended message. In a man–computer system, a third phase is added. The verbalized human ideas must be transformed into machine-compatible symbols. The machine has to handle natural language. Moreover, the machine must "understand" the human communication, and then generate the information according to the user's needs. The problem is at the man–machine interface, at the computer terminals. The medical communication must be entered, via the terminal, and the natural language communication must be transformed into computer-compatible language. A paralanguage is needed, which is a high-fidelity translation of the human language into computer-oriented codes. This paralanguage must conserve the semantic content of the medical communication. Once the input is converted into the paralanguage, the next task is to "teach" the computer to "understand" the ideas expressed by the human communication. Further, a vast storage space is necessary for the medical knowledge. Based upon the input, the machine should "understand" the physician's information needs, fetch the pertinent information from the data base, and display them for the physician. This information display must be in human-compatible natural language. The man–machine interaction must be rapid, to enable the user to carry out a dialogue as if the machine were a human expert answering questions.

The purpose of this rather primitive summary of the man–machine system is to identify the component tasks, which include:

1. Transformation of the natural language medical text into a semantically equivalent paralanguage.
2. Degradation, semantically, of the submitted information for a logical perception ("understanding") of medical text so that the human communication is appercepted by the machine. (In this context, apperception is the transcendental integration of information into the machine-stored cohesive information base. In simpler words, the machine must unbundle and liberate the implicit semantic content attached to the medical text.)
3. Building a large, comprehensive data base containing a patient data bank and medical knowledge bank.
4. Constructing computer programs that can carry out the requests of the users of the terminal (viz., to accept, store, or retrieve needed information).

THE PARALANGUAGE OF MEDICINE

Computational linguistics is the scientific discipline focusing on the analysis of the natural language, in order to represent human communication in the computer. Linguistics separates natural language into two component forces: semantics and syntax. Semantics is the theory of reference (denotation and extension) and the theory of meaning. Syntax is the set of rules, the grammar of the natural language. Formulating the sentence, the structural unit of the natural language requires syntactic grammar. The rules of grammar are very complex, but they enable us to make infinite use of a finite number of words.

In our program, we limited our paralanguage strictly to the semantic representation of the medical communication. We built a paralanguage as a semantic mirror image of the human language. This paralanguage is, in fact, an open-ended list of codes, where each code represents one entity (i.e., one word or term of the natural language). A medical statement is a string of words or terms in the human language and an equal number of codes in the paralanguage. This paralanguage consists of: (a) medical terms, representing medical ideas, and (b) "cement" words, which are nonmedical (i.e., "before," "was," "above," "next").

The tool for transforming a medical text into such a paralanguage is the medical lexicon, where we compile the human words and their paralanguage equivalents. The terms and words in this lexicon can be ordered in an alphabetic sequence. This facilitates finding a needed entry. The role of the medical lexicon is somewhat similar to that of the telephone directory, which lists the subscribers in alphabetic sequence, followed by the telephone system's code. By dialing the code, we can reach the subscriber.

The computer-oriented medical lexicon is the bridge between the human verbalization (natural language) and the machine-oriented code scheme (paralanguage). The lexicon must be comprehensive, in order to handle any word that may occur in a medical text. It must be semantically cross-referenced to indicate semantic relatedness and controlled in order to keep each lexical entry unique (rule of mutual exclusiveness).

A lexical entry may be a single word or a group of words representing a single distinct medical idea, for example, [acute appendicitis] or [acute viral hepatitis, type B].

The code attached to each lexical entry is unique so that a one-to-one relationship exists between the lexical entry and its code. For cross-referencing purposes, a string of semantic codes is attached to the unique code. These semantic codes range from synonymy to more distant semantic relatedness (superterms, lateral terms, and subterms) so that each lexical term is inserted into a cohesive semantic system. These codes will be discussed further in a later part of this paper.

AUTOMATED ENCODING

Upon submission of a medical text, a program decomposes the text and finds the corresponding lexical entries in the lexicon. This search calls for a letter-by-letter match. When a successful match is accomplished, the program substitutes the natural language word(s) for a string of paralanguage codes. In reality, this transformation is a complex technical process, but the result of the actual transformation is obvious. The natural language words are transformed, without any semantic/syntactic changes, into an equivalent paralanguage. This design enabled us to type in a medical text and make it computer-compatible by a single, rapid, simple operation.

The automated encoding process transforms the input text into the paralanguage. The opposite process takes place as a last step before the display of a computer output. The program converts the paralanguage into natural language, for human use. This is automated decoding.

THE DATA BANKS

PRAKTICE (*P*hysicians' *R*ecords *a*nd *K*nowledge yielding *T*otal *I*nformation *C*onsulted *E*lectronically) is the collective name of our medical information system. The first component of PRAKTICE, the Medical Lexicon, was briefly described above. The major part of PRAKTICE is, however, composed of four separate but integrated data banks. This design reflects the basic assumption outlined above, that the physician needs four types of information in his clinical work: (1) past history of the patient; (2) clinical experience in similar cases; (3) pertinent sections of the appropriate textbooks; and (4) pertinent research activities. Possessing these four types of pertinent information, the clinician should be able to make the "best" (scientifically optimized) decisions in diagnosis and therapy.

The Clinical Case History Bank

Input: Medical Records. This data bank was designed to store and retrieve individual patients' past medical histories. In this bank, for each patient a file is created, and this file is updated when a new clinical event is submitted. A clinical event may be an office visit or a hospitalization episode. This way, the patient files are longitudinal and cumulative.

The data source for this data bank is the physician's record (viz., the hospital discharge record or the office record). We enter, word by word, everything the physician has recorded. The submitted record is automatically encoded, with the assistance of the Medical Lexicon, and the medical record, in paralanguage, is subsequently added to the file of the appropriate patient.

Entering the medical record in the PRAKTICE system is simply a matter of keying in the physician's notes. The data entry clerks soon learn how to interpret the typical medical abbreviations, and then the entry is expeditious.

For the protection of the confidentiality of the clinical data, the patient identifiers are stored in a separate file, the physician/institution identifiers in a second file, and the actual clinical data in a third file. These three files can be linked only via an "authorization program." This authorization program can be invoked routinely only when the attending physician requests the display of his patient's history, in his office, during his customary office hours.

Outputs. *Case Summaries.* As the patient's file increases, it is not practical to present the entire file to the clinician. As time passes, many data become less important, and the physician needs the case summary rather than the retrieval of the entire record. We have designed two types of case summaries. The Synopsis is a very brief summary, whereas the Extended Case Summary contains more details.

The Synopsis is assembled algorithmically:

This is a . . . . year old (white/black) (male/female), on file since . . . . . .
Diagnoses: (diagnoses and date) . . . . . . Surgeries . . . . Allergies . . . . . .
Last visit for (diagnosis) was on . . . . Current drug therapy . . . .

The Extended Case Summary also includes all significant abnormal laboratory, X-ray data, and other diagnostic findings and a table of dates of all past clinical events with the diagnoses.

Patient Files. If the clinician needs the full record rather than the Synopsis or the Extended Case Summary, PRAKTICE can readily retrieve the entire file.

The Clinical Case History Bank consists of three major files:

1. *The patient identifiers* (e.g., name, address, telephone number, referred by, insurance carrier, fiscal history, next scheduled visit, and internal code number).
2. *The physician/institution identifiers* with the internal code number.
3. *Clinical data* under the internal code number.

These three sets of data on the same patient can be linked together by means of the code number. The patient's date of birth is the verifying information kept in all three files. The purpose of this verifying information is to confirm the correctness of the internal code number.

The Clinical Data Bank consists of all the individual patient files kept in chronologic sequence. At the end of the patient's file is the Synopsis and the Extended Case Summary. After the filing of a clinical event, the Synopsis and the Extended Case Summary are automatically updated.

Billing and Scheduling. Since the data elements of patient billing are captured (patient identifiers, insurance carriers, service provider, diagnosis, and services rendered), PRAKTICE can provide automated billing. Patient scheduling is another capability of PRAKTICE.

Clinical Experience Bank

This bank is the storage of statistical data derived from the Clinical Case History Bank. Whereas the latter is organized by patient, the Clinical Experience Bank is the summary by clinical features (e.g., diagnoses, therapy, clinical course, epidemiologic parameters).

The diagnostic files list the number of cases with exactly the same diagnosis and the number of cases with very similar diagnoses. The user of the system can see from these data the frequency of occurrence of such a diagnosis, or the user may request the related therapy data. Such a statistical report shows how cases with that particular diagnosis were treated by others. The user may also ask for the apparent success rate of the various therapeutic alternatives, or he may ask for clinical manifestations (signs and symptoms, diagnostic studies), or the clinical course. Thus, the Clinical Experience Bank is a prepared set of statistical analyses. The user may ask not only for similar cases, but also for all cases receiving the same drug, or all cases with similar signs and symptoms.

The epidemiologic statistics are conceived within the geographic structure as a time-related statistics.

The clinical data, as well as the therapeutic data, are extensively classified and systematized in the Clinical Experience Bank. This way, the user can request exact correspondence (e.g., patients who meet all the search criteria such as age, family history, and diagnosis), near-correspondence (all cases of bronchogenic carcinoma), or similar cases (all cases of osteoporosis). For such a flexibility of information retrieval, extensive semantic cross-referencing of the clinical data is necessary. In PRAKTICE, this capability is built into the Medical Lexicon. Classification will be discussed further in the next section of this chapter.

Knowledge Bank

At the outset, the goal of PRAKTICE was to provide the user with pertinent information. This calls for an interactive dialogue capability, and the computer is expected to "understand" the medical terms. Transforming a natural language term into its paralanguage is only a first step. Then, the computer must be able to pass the terms through a cognitive process to "understand" them. For example, when the computer receives the term "hepatitis," it should "know" that this is a nonspecific classifying term covering [viral hepatitis], [alcoholic hepatitis], [drug-induced hepatitis], etc. Medical terms carry a varying amount of implicit information, and the computer must be able to "unbundle" this implicit information.

In interhuman communication, the receiver's first step is the recognition of the words. The second step is a cognitive processing. When a physician receives a medical message, it is promptly related to the pertinent knowledge preexisting in his memory. This associative information processing places the received message into a medical context essential for full perception.

To illustrate this complex mental process, let us consider the following warning message:

$$\left\{ \text{Drug X may cause hepatitis.} \right\}$$

The initial perceptive process separates the warning into its components: (a) [Drug X] (b) (may cause) (c) [hepatitis]. The target term in this message is [hepatitis] and the recipient must process, cognitively, this term for a full understanding of the message. First, the physician "knows" the implicit meaning of [hepatitis] as:

— diffuse liver damage;
— causing malaise, jaundice;
— diagnosable with liver tests.

The physician also knows the usual clinical course of such "drug-induced" hepatitis.

Our task is to deposit medical knowledge, in an organized manner, into the computer, as an artificial medical memory where [hepatitis] can be "decoded" semantically by the machine. This calls for an organized cognitive matrix that represents current medical knowledge.

We have studied extensively the ways the physician builds up his own cognitive memory. In the medical school, this is preplanned by the curriculum committee. The first year of the medical school begins with courses in anatomy and histology. The student must first memorize the normal structures of the human body. At the end of this period, the student "knows" the normal structures of the human body as well as their normal functions. After learning "basic sciences," the student is exposed to clinical sciences. Tutorial learning of a disease is often reinforced by first referring to normal structures/functions. This helps the student to build up the cognitive pathways in his medical cognitive memory.

In order to reconstruct this human learning process, we considered the artificial cognitive memory as a set of nodes (terms) with connecting arcs. These arcs represent relationships among the nodes. There are some nodes that require little or no cognitive processing, such as [liver] or [heart], whereas others must undergo a series of steps that represent the cognitive processing. In order to structure this process, in PRAKTICE we have divided the medical terms into seven categories (see chart).

VII	THEORIES — HEALTH SERVICES
VI	TREATMENTS
V	ETIOLOGY
IV	DISEASES
III	MEASUREMENTS
II	NORMAL FUNCTIONS
I	NORMAL STRUCTURES

These seven categories (classes) reflect the extent of cognitive processing required for understanding a medical term. Terms in the first class require no processing, whereas a higher-class term depends on the support of the lower classes. If we use the example above, [hepatitis], we can follow the process of cognition:

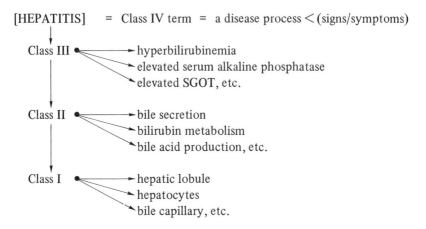

[HEPATITIS] = Class IV term = a disease process < (signs/symptoms)

Class III → hyperbilirubinemia
elevated serum alkaline phosphatase
elevated SGOT, etc.

Class II → bile secretion
bilirubin metabolism
bile acid production, etc.

Class I → hepatic lobule
hepatocytes
bile capillary, etc.

Thus, the cognitive cascade of arcs from the origin [hepatitis] leads to lower-level terms that are semantically implicit in the higher-level term. The physician "knows" what [hepatitis] means, and the semantic cascade of arcs enables the machine to know it. These arcs unbundle the semantic content of the higher-level medical term.

Perhaps the most difficult medical task encountered during the construction of PRAKTICE was to develop these arcs and nodes representing formalized medical knowledge. Very briefly, our medical knowledge is a composite of atomic facts. These facts must meet certain criteria:

A fact must be *true*: [A (always, often, sometimes, never) causes B].

A fact must be *medically significant* (it may affect a clinical decision such as diagnosis, therapy, prognosis).

A fact must be *integrated* (with other closely related facts).

A fact must be *unique* (represented only once in the cognitive memory).

A fact must be *explicitly* represented (free of ambiguity, as accurate as available knowledge permits).

A fact must be *contiguous* (direct semantic attachment to a preceding and a subsequent statement, without information gaps).

A fact must be *consistent* with the corpus of facts in the data bank.

Classification of the medical terms into the seven classes gave us some further insights. If a word is a medical term, it is also a node, with a cluster of arcs connecting the node with other nodes. If a node is an anatomic term, such as [thyroid] or [tibia], it has a definitional arc [thyroid = an endocrine gland, tibia = a bone], where the arcs relate the term to its superterm:

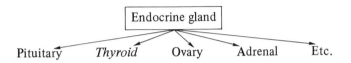

Another group of arcs lead to subterms covered by the node:

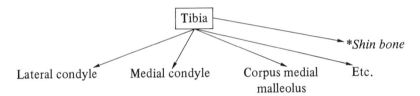

* = synonym; the other arcs lead to the subterms.

Other arcs connect the anatomic node with its specific *histologic* and *subcellular* ultrastructural components. Still other arcs represent topographic relatedness; for example, [liver]   [diaphragm], and there are arcs indicating embryologic/developmental relationships.

As we move from anatomic nodes to higher-level nodes, the cluster of arcs changes, as, for example, a IV-level term such as [gout] carries the following arcs:

1. Definition arc (Class IV term = disturbance of purine metabolism)
2. Clinical history/symptoms arcs – typical complaints
3. Clinical signs arcs
4. Differential diagnostic arcs
5. Diagnostic study arcs (laboratory, X-rays, etc.)
6. Pathochemical arcs – xanthine metabolic disturbances
7. Genetic arcs (autosomal dominant, polygenic)
8. Clinical course arcs
9. Therapy arcs
10. Epidemiologic arcs

The cluster of typical arcs is different if a node belongs to Category VI. For example, a drug has the following arcs:

1. Name = chemical definition, generic
2. Manufacturer(s) — if applicable brand product and/or combination drug
3. Clinical pharmacology data including pharmacogenetics
4. Pharmacokinetic data
5. Indications for administering the durg
6. Contraindications
7. Use in pregnancy
8. Warning
9. Drug interactions (with other drugs)
10. Drug interference (with laboratory tests)
11. Toxic effects
12. Treatment of toxicity

This design of nodes and arcs ultimately results in a medical cognitive network. Any note may be addressed directly, through the Medical Lexicon, and all connecting arcs also can be used for information acquisition, in an interactive mode.

Biomedical Research Bank

Whereas the other capabilities of PRAKTICE have been extensively field-tested, the Biomedical Research Bank underwent only a technical field-testing to demonstrate its feasibility and to check the cost of maintaining such an information service.

The Biomedical Research Bank consists of a Block Directory and blocks. Each block contains one research report 4-7 condensed into the following sections:

1. *The Message:* A brief but succinct summary of the study, if possible in one sentence.
2. *The Model:* The chosen parameters and measured variables. If an animal model is used, the selection of the experimental animals is also a part of the section.
3. *Procedure:* The study.
4. *Findings:* The interpretation of the results.
5. *Evaluation:* An expert reviewer's opinion about the level of credibility of the study expressed numerically on a scale of 0 to 10. A well-documented paper would receive a value of 10, whereas at the other end of the scale, a very low value should be given to an entirely speculative paper lacking any confirming evidence.
6. *References:* This section contains the bibliographic identifiers such as: author(s), title of paper/monograph/book, language (English, German, etc.), name of journal or publisher, name of reviewer.

All the contents of the first four sections are in paralanguage, using the Medical Lexicon. Therefore, pertinent literature can be retrieved by searching for the pertinent key words (= medical terms) in the Block Directory.

QUESTION-ANSWERING CAPABILITY

PRAKTICE was designed to provide the medical users with all the necessary information for optimized information-dependent decisions. Accordingly, the system can provide:

1. The patient's past medical history (or a synopsis or extended case history).
2. Pertinent clinical experience (in cases with similar signs/symptoms, in cases with similar diagnosis, in cases receiving the same drug therapy, etc.).
3. Pertinent sections of the knowledge bank.
4. Pertinent research findings.

These four types of capabilities of PRAKTICE should enable the clinician to optimize his information-dependent decisions. The overall flow of steps is as follows:

1. *User:* States information need (patient record, experience, knowledge, or research).
2. *PRAKTICE:* Transforms information into paralanguage.
3. *PRAKTICE:* "Understands" the information need of the user.
4. *PRAKTICE:* Retrieves the information requested.
5. *User:* If the retrieved information prompted the user to ask for further information, a second cycle of 1 through 4 is carried out, and the dialogue is continued until the user is satisfied.

This question-answering capability of our PRAKTICE system is important for the physician using the system. Other capabilities such as automated billing and scheduling make PRAKTICE a highly cost-effective information system.

MEMORIZABLE VS. COMPUTABLE MEDICAL KNOWLEDGE

Concerned about the growing information deficit, academic medicine should recognize that computer technology can solve the problem of our acute information overload. Instead of further reduction of the practical content of the medical school curriculum, an entirely new approach is needed. First, a painstaking study will be necessary to separate the present medical school curriculum into two components: memorizable knowledge, which is still essential and required for a physician to function (with the assistance of a computer), and computable knowledge, which can be stored/retrieved when needed. A surgeon could hardly operate with confidence without good working knowledge in surgical anatomy, but the selection of the "best" surgical procedure may be computed if such a decision calls for experience data.

If we critically examined vast areas that, by default, we memorize today, such as biochemistry or pharmacology or genetics, we could begin to develop *quantitative aspects* of the matter. In a recent edition of the *Textbook of Medicine,*[2] the chapter on diseases of the bone, with 22 sections, contains 94 facts on bone physiology and 1114 hard clinical facts on 42 diseases.

A recent monograph on inherited disorders of the skeleton[7] lists 120 clinical entities instead of the 14 diseases described by Beeson and McDermott.[2]

If we further pursue this line of reasoning, we will readily find additional quantitative data. For example, the disease [osteogenesis imperfecta] has the following representations:

In the *Textbook of Medicine*, 36 hard facts are listed under osteogenesis imperfecta; in the monograph on hereditary bone disorders 47 additional facts are given; and after an extensive library search extracting an additional 68 more or less hard facts, we can assume total knowledge in this particular area to be about 151 data.

As computer technology evolves, storage and retrieval of medical data is less and less expensive. A single national medical knowledge bank could support all practitioners in the United States, to any preset level of specificity; at the level of textbooks or monographs, or covering the newest research reports as well.

Academic medicine may rethink medical education in terms of computable vs. memorizable medical knowledge. Perhaps directed studies should be initiated to separate essential knowledge in internal medicine, surgery, or obstetrics from computable information. We believe such an approach would reduce the present medical school curriculum by 75-80%. Thus, the residual essential memorizable material could be expanded to produce better physicians.

Perhaps the selection of the medical students should also be revised. It is quite apparent that college grades are not sufficiently accurate for identifying the good physician candidates of the future. Excellent memorizers may not be the most dedicated candidates for medical schools. Interest in helping others, empathy, and commitment should receive more attention. Moreover, in a man-machine system, rational decision-making, crisp logic, sharp reasoning, and humanitarian interests are the highest values. Our present admission policies are not tailored to this set of values.

SUMMARY

PRAKTICE is a concept, as well as an aggregate of computer programs, transferring computable data to a computer. The physician-user of PRAKTICE receives four types of data from the computer, as an interactive consultation: (1) the patient's past medical history; (2) pertinent clinical experience; (3) pertinent formal knowledge; and (4) pertinent research data. PRAKTICE accepts natural language input, processes data in a medical paralanguage, and "understands" medical terms. The impact of such a computer-assisted clinical system upon the practice of medicine and medical education is briefly discussed.

REFERENCES

1. Anderson, W. A. D., and J. M. Kissane (eds.): *Pathology*, 7th ed. St. Louis: C. V. Mosby, 1977.
2. Beeson, Paul B., and W. McDermott: *Textbook of Medicine*, 14th ed. Philadelphia: Saunders, 1955.
3. Gabrieli, E. R.: *Advanced Uses of Information Processing Technology In Clinical Medicine*. American Society of Clinical Pathologists, 1979.
4. Gabrieli, E. R.: "Medical Information System, Health Records and Knowledge Banks." *Med. Instru.* 12:245, 1978.
5. Gabrieli, E. R.: "Computerization of Information on RES." *J. RES* 8:349, 1970.
6. Gabrieli, E. R.: "Programming a Medical Information System." *J. Clin. Computing* 7:25, 1977.
7. Beighton, P.: *Inherited Disorders of the Skeleton*. Edinburgh: Churchill Livingstone, 1978.

5
MEDICAL PRIVACY AND CONFIDENTIALITY

George J. Annas, J.D., M.P.H.
Associate Professor of Law and Medicine
Department of Socio-Medical Sciences and
Community Medicine, Boston University
Schools of Medicine and Public Health

The more dependent society becomes upon the maintenance of a galaxy of information systems, the more defined two conflicting trends become. The first, exemplified by state and federal "freedom of information" of "sunshine" acts, aims at providing the public access to all information held by governmental agencies. The permise is that public knowledge of the most intimate details of how government works is likely to make government more responsive to the will of the people and also prevent official wrongdoing. The second is exemplified by state and federal laws aimed at protecting information about individual citizens from public disclosure. While details remain to be worked out in many areas, the consensus is that with all forms of personal-data-keeping systems — credit, insurance, education, taxation, criminal, and medical, to name some of the most important — individuals have or should have a right of "privacy" broad enough to enable them to examine and correct the information and to prevent the release of this information without their express consent.

Medical records have been the last to come under public scrutiny, perhaps because medicine has a tradition of "keeping confidences." Nevertheless, as the solo practitioner-patient relationship becomes an endangered species, record keeping in medicine comes to resemble other massive record-keeping systems. Accordingly, the rules applied to these systems are likely to become applicable to medical records as well. As to medical records specifically, there have only been a couple of dozen cases that have reached the appellate courts. The law in this area must therefore be considered to be in its infancy, and resort must often be made to public policy and arguments by analogy.

This chapter will focus on the legal concepts of privacy and confidentiality, the exceptions to these doctrines, and the considerations that should go into a decision about releasing confidential medical information to anyone but the patient. It will be noted that computerization of medical records does not change the nature of the major legal issues involved, but does make some of them more immediately compelling.

DEFINITIONS

Almost all of the existing law concerning third-party access to medical records can be placed under the headings of confidentiality, privilege, and privacy. In common usage, to tell someone something in confidence means that the person will not repeat what was said to anyone. Confidentiality thus presupposes that something "secret" will be told to someone. The presumption is that the secret will not be repeated. Relationships such as attorney-client, priest–penitent, and doctor-patient are confidential relationships. In the doctor-patient context, confidentiality is descriptive of an express or implied agreement that the doctor will not disclose the information received from the patient to anyone not directly involved in the patient's care and treatment.

A communication is said to be privileged if the person to whom the information is given is forbidden by law from disclosing it in a court proceeding without the consent of the person who provided it. Privilege is a legal rule of evidence, applying only in the judicial context. Moreover, the privilege belongs to the client, not to the professional. Unlike the attorney-client privilege, the doctor-patient privilege is not recognized at common law, and therefore exists only in those states that have passed a statute establishing it. Fewer than a dozen states have no such statute regarding physicians.

There at least two senses in which the term privacy is generally used. The first describes a constitutional right of privacy. This right, while not found directly enunciated in the Constitution, was the basis for decisions by the U. S. Supreme Court limiting state interference with birth control and abortion. This right is said to be one of personal privacy and involves the ability of an individual to make important, intimate decisions.

In the more traditional sense the term has been defined as "the right to be let alone, to be free of prying, peeping, and snooping," and as "the right of someone to keep information about himself or access to his personality inaccessible to others."[1]

LAW AND ETHICS

The maintenance of confidentiality is both a legal and an ethical obligation of health-care providers. Historically the doctrine was an ethical duty applicable only to physicians. Currently it is also a legal duty of physicians (as enunciated in case law, and some state licensing statutes), and it is becoming a legal duty of other health-care practitioners as well.

The Hippocratic Oath first set out the duty of confidentiality in the following words:

> Whatsoever things I see or hear concerning the life of man, in any attendance on the sick or even apart therefrom which ought not to be noised about, I will keep silent thereon, counting such things to be professional secrets.

This oath has been reinterpreted in the current formulation of the American Medical Association's Principles of Ethics:

> A physician may not reveal the confidences entrusted to him in the course of medical attendance, or the deficiencies he may observe in the character of patients, unless he is required to do so by law or unless it becomes necessary in order to protect the welfare of the individual or the community.

Similarly, Section 2 of the American Nurses' Association Code provides: "The nurse safeguards the client's right to privacy by judiciously protecting information of a confidential nature." The interpretative statements elaborate:

> When knowlege gained in confidence is relevant or essential to others involved in planning or implementing the client's care, professional judgment is used in sharing it. Only information pertinent to a client's treatment and welfare is disclosed and only to those directly concerned with the client's care .... The nurse–client relationship is built on trust. This relationship could be destroyed and the client's welfare and reputation jeopardized by injudicious disclosure of information provided in confidence.

The reason for all of these rules, of course, is that health-care providers need to know the most personal and possibly embarrassing details of the patient's life to help the patient, and patients are not likely to freely disclose these details unless they are certain that no one else, not directly involved in their care, will learn of them. As one court described the patient's dilemma:

> Since a layman is unfamiliar with the road to recovery, he cannot sift the circumstances of his life and habits to determine what is information pertinent to his health. As a consequence, he must disclose all information in his consultations with his doctor — even that which is embarrassing, disgraceful, or incriminating. To promote full disclosure, the medical profession extends the

promise of secrecy. The candor which this promise elicits is necessary to the effective pursuit of health; there can be no reticence, no reservation, no reluctance when patients discuss their problems with their doctors.[2]

THE COURTS

Even though the law is quite explicit, it is notable that there are few reported cases involving breaches of confidentiality. This can mean that such violations are rare, patients never learn of violations when they do occur, patients don't think it is appropriate to sue for such violations (because of the cost, uncertain damages, and possible further publicity of the confidential information), or almost all such cases are settled before they reach an appellate court.

Those cases that have been appealed have most often alleged violation of confidences by physicians in one of the following situations: disclosure to a spouse (involving either a disease related to the marriage or a condition relevant in a divorce, alimony, or custody action), disclosure to an insurance company, or disclosure to an employer.[3]

Also, in court proceedings, the privilege doctrine applies. There are two competing values in this doctrine. The first is that certain types of relationships are potentially so beneficial to individuals and society that they should be fostered by forbidding in-court disclosure of the informational content of the relationship. A privilege is therefore granted to encourage the employment of professionals by individuals who need their services and to promote absolute freedom of communication. The contrary principle is that the courtroom is a place for the discovery of truth, and no reliable source of truth should be beyond the reach of the court. At common law the court's interest in the truth routinely won out, and physicians were forced to testify to the matters disclosed to them by their patients.

The great majority of courts currently agree that the principal reason for the privilege is to encourage a patient to freely and frankly reveal to his physician all the facts and symptoms concerning his condition so that the physician will be in the best possible position to correctly diagnose and successfully treat the patient, and most states have adopted the privilege by statute. Nevertheless, the statutory adoption of the privilege was strongly criticized by John Henry Wigmore, late dean of Northwestern University Law School and perhaps the authority on the law of evidence. He argued that in most cases it only serves to frustrate the ends of justice by denying truthful information to courts. He contended, for example, that most information communicated to a physician is not intended to be held strictly confidential, since most of one's ailments are both immediately apparent and openly discussed; and that even when information is intended to be maintained as confidential, it would be disclosed to the physician even if no privilege existed. Finally he noted that in litigation involving personal injuries it is absurd that the physician not be required to disclose the true extent of the litigant's injuries.[4]

THE "RIGHT OF PRIVACY"

In his book *Privacy and Freedom,* Alan Westin defines privacy as "the claim of individuals, groups, or institutions to determine for themselves when, how, and to what extent information about them is communicated to others."[5] He goes on to argue that, as thus defined, the concept has its roots in the territorial behavior of animals, and its importance can be seen to some extent throughout the history of civilization. Specific protections of privacy were built into the U. S. Constitution by the framers in terms that were important to their government. With the subsequent inventions of the telephone, radio, television, and computer systems, more sophisticated legal doctrines were developed in an attempt to protect the informational privacy of the individual.

One such approach was suggested by Warren and Brandeis in the *Harvard Law Review* in 1890. Their approach, directed toward private rather than public or governmental invasions, suggested that there be developed a legal remedy for individuals whose privacy was invaded by the press or others for commercial gain. As a result of this and other arguments, a number of states passed statutes making such invasions actionable at law. While many diverse acts may be said to come under the heading of privacy violations that may give rise to a cause of action, most involving medical records would fall in the area generally described as the "publication [disclosing to one or more unauthorized person] of private matters violating ordinary decencies."

A court can find the unauthorized disclosure of medical records an actionable invasion of privacy even without a state statute that specifically forbids it. As an Alabama court put it in a case involving disclosure of medical information to a patient's employer:

> Unauthorized disclosure of intimate details of a patient's health may amount to unwarranted publication of one's private affaris with which the public has no legitimate concern such as to cause outrage, mental suffering, shame, or humiliation to a person of ordinary sensibilities.[6]

The policy underlying the right is that certain information about individuals should not be repeated without their permission. In the words of one legal commentator: "The basic attribute of an effective right to privacy is the individual's ability to control the flow of information concerning or describing him."[7] Most of the cases in the doctor-patient context alleging violation of the right to privacy have involved actions in which personal medical information has been published in a newspaper or magazine, and often the suit is against the publisher rather than the physician.[8]

EXCEPTIONS TO CONFIDENTIALITY

Mandatory Disclosures

While the doctines of confidentiality and privacy are, on the surface, very powerful legal tools, their effect in the day-to-day practice of medicine is considerably diluted by the exceptions and defenses physicians and other health-care providers can raise to a charge of unauthorized disclosure. There have been no reported appellate decision in the United States, for example, in which any health-care provider or hospital has ever had to pay money damages to a patient for the unauthorized disclosure of medical information. Indeed, there are situations in which health-care professionals *must* disclose confidential information, even though they may not want to:

1. Public Reporting Statutes. Almost all states have a wide variety of conditions and diseases that must be reported to the public authorities when discovered by the physician. These fall into four major categories: vital statistics, contagious and dangerous diseases, child neglect and abuse, and criminally inflicted injuries. All decree a public policy that takes precedence over the health-care professional's obligation to maintain a patient's confidences.

(a) In the first category are birth and death certificates. In the case of birth certificates, information on the parents is generally required. If death is from an accidental cause, sudden, or foul play is suspected, the medical examiner or coroner is usually required by law to perform an autopsy and file a complete report of his findings with the district attorney. These reporting statutes are almost universally complied with, and failure to do so is generally a misdemeanor punishable by both fine and imprisonment.

(b) Typical infectious, contagious, or communicable diseases that must be reported are listed in the California statute as: cholera, plague, yellow fever, malaria, leprosy, diphtheria, scarlet fever, smallpox, typhus fever, typhoid fever, paratyphoid fever, anthrax, glanders, epidemic cerebrospinal meningitis, tuberculosis, pneumonia, dysentery, erysipelas, hookworm, trachoma, dengue, tetanus, measles, German measles, chickenpox, whooping cough, mumps, pellagra, beriberi, Rocky Mountain spotted fever, syphilis, gonorrhea, rabies, or poliomyelitis.[9] Most public health officials agree that only a fraction of many of these diseases are reported by physicians, and this is a major problem.

(c) Reporting of child abuse cases is generally limited to the emergency rooms of large city hospitals. A recent California case, however, concluded that a physician could be held liable to pay damages suffered by a child whose parents seriously abused her after the physician had treated her for a previous injury resulting from abuse that he did not report.[10] Failure to report can also subject a health professional to criminal penalties, and this obligation should be taken extremely seriously so that children can be protected from abusive custodians.

(d) The final category includes things like "a bullet wound, gunshot wound, powder burn or any other injury arising from or caused by the discharge of a gun or firearm, and every case of a wound which is likely to or may result in death and is actually or apparently inflicted by a knife, icepick or other sharp instrument."[11]

2. Judicial Process. When someone makes his own physical condition an issue in a lawsuit (e.g., a personal injury claim), most courts will permit examination of his physician under oath either before or during the trial. Even in states that have privilege statutes, there are generally many exceptions that would permit bringing medical information into court. For example, medical information is often available in criminal cases, and almost always in malpractice cases. When a judge requires a health-care provider to disclose confidential information in a judicial proceeding, the provider must comply or face a penalty for contempt of court.

3. Federal and State Statutes Concerning Cost and Quality Control. There are a variety of state and federal statutes that permit certain monitoring agencies to have access to patient charts for such purposes as peer review, utilization review, studies to protect against provider reimbursement fraud, and licensing and accreditation surveys. The most pervasive of these statutes is the federal statute and regulations on Professional Standards Review Organizations. Current regulations require that the information collected under this program not be made public in any way in which individual practitioners or patients can be identified.

4. Patient Who Poses a Danger to Known Third Party. Until very recently, physicians have only been held responsible for injuries inflicted on others by their patients when they were directly negligent in their treatment of the patient. For example, physicians have been held responsible for negligently failing to diagnose TB, thereby placing family members at risk;[12] for wrongly informing a patient's neighbor that smallpox was not contagious;[13] and for wrongly informing the members of a family that typhoid fever[14] and scarlet fever[15] of a sibling would not infect other members of the family.

The California Supreme Court recently went somewhat further than this, ruling that: "When a doctor or a psychotherapist, in the exercise of his professional skill and knowledge, determines, or *should determine,* that a warning is essential to avert danger arising from the medical or psychological condition of his patient, he incurs a *legal obligation* to give that warning."[16] The case involved a patient who had threatened to kill his former girlfriend. The therapist believed him, took some initial steps to have him confined, and then, allegedly on orders from his superior, dropped the case. The patient in fact killed the young woman, and her family sued the therapist. The California Supreme Court declared, in the above-quoted language, that the therapist could be found liable. The case was eventually settled out of court.

The psychiatric profession argued vehemently against this ruling, saying it would curtail the ability of psychiatrists to treat patients who would not come to them because they feared being reported to the authorities, and would encourage psychiatrists to have potentially dangerous patients committed to mental institutions rather than take a chance of continuing to treat them on an out-patient basis.[17] However one comes out on this individual practitioner right vs. the rights of society question, it must be recognized by all that the broader we as a society make the health-care professional's mandate to report his patient's condition to others, the more like a policeman the health-care professional becomes. Nevertheless, health-care providers have an obligation to society as well as to their patients. When the life of another can be saved by breaching a confidence, and there is no reasonable alternative to accomplishing the same objective, courts (and society in general) will have little difficulty in mandating disclosure.

The question of what obligation, if any, the *custodian* of medical records should have to make reports has never been raised, but computerization at least makes retrieval of relevant information easier and may lead to demands for certain types of reports to public agencies.

Optional Disclosure

The "optional" disclosure situations are extremely broad, and indicate the vast discretion courts are likely to afford health-care professionals acting in good faith:

1. Implied Consent. This is probably the major cause of leakage from the current medical records system. When a patient is in a hospital, for example, he by implication consents to the viewing of his medical record by all those directly concerned with his care. This may include the nurses on all three shifts, the ward secretary, all medical students, interns, and residents in the hospital, the attending physician and any consultants called in, and perhaps social, psychological, medical, or psychiatric researchers. All of this may take place without the patient's being made aware of it, and it is said to be a matter of custom.

2. General Release Forms (Consent). Upon entering a hospital a patient may be asked to sign a wide variety of forms. One of these forms is likely to be an authorization saying essentially that the hospital may release medical information concerning the patient to anyone it thinks should have it or to certain named agencies or organizations. This will include such persons as insurance companies, the welfare department (if they are paying all or part of the bill), and other agencies or individuals monitoring cost. No restriction is generally placed on the amount of material that may be released or the use to which many of these third parties may put the information so received. Arguably, however, receivers would be liable for an invasion-of-privacy action if they used the medical information for other than the specific purpose for which the hospital released it.

Although I am not aware of the argument's ever having been made, it would seem that most these general release forms could be attacked as unduly broad and so vague that the patient could not reasonably and knowingly have signed them. The cases regarding the invalidity of blanket surgical consent forms, which give the doctor and hospital authority to perform whatever procedures they think necessary, would support this line of reasoning. Another argument that could be made is that the patient's lack of bargaining power made the form ineffective (e.g., a sick patient may need admission and cannot afford to forgo it by refusing to sign a required form).[18]

3. Private Interests of the Patient. Courts seem to afford physicians generous latitude in making disclosures that physicians believe in good faith are in the best interests of their patients. This rule, for example, is used to justify many disclosures to spouses and near relatives without the patient's consent. While this practice has been criticized on the grounds that when only the patient's individual welfare is involved, only the patient should have the right to decide when confidential information should be released,[19] courts will probably continue to give physicians and hospitals much discretion in this area, so long as they can make a reasonable argument that there were no alternatives available and the patient's own health required the disclosure.

Even though there has been little judicial explanation of the content of this exception, one can deduce that such cases as telling a spouse of a patient's heart condition or impending death, or telling an employer of a roofer that the roofer is subject to blackouts (since the patient would be endangering his own life by continuing in this trade), would probably qualify.

Those in charge of the computer that processes medical data will need clear rules on the circumstances under which "optional" data — with or without personal identifiers — can be released.

PUBLIC CONCERN ABOUT COMPUTERIZED MEDICAL RECORDS

Although most of the evidence on this question is anecdotal, there seems to be little doubt that patients would prefer to see confidential medical information shared with as few people as possible. A study that tends to confirm this was conducted in Georgia in 1974-75.[20] In July 1974, the mental health clinics and centers in the state of Georgia were required to send personal information on individual clients to the state capitol. Patients were asked to sign the following release form:

> The undersigned patient hereby authorizes the Northeast Georgia Community Mental Health Center to furnish the Division of Mental Health of the Georgia Department of Human Resources a record or records including the following information: patient's name, social security number, and nature of patient's primary disability.

A final clause provided that the information would not be made publicly available. Of 962 clients at the Center's four clinics, no one refused to sign.

From March to September of 1975, Dr. Catherine E. Rosen used two alternative procedures. The same form was used, but in two of the four clinics after reading it the client was informed orally that if he signed, this information would be placed in the Mental Health computer file. In the other two clinics, this statement was followed by another: "If you do not sign this paper, this identifying information will not be sent into the state offices in the capitol and will be kept only locally. In other words, if you don't sign you will get the same services from us as if you did sign."

In the two clinics where only the first "no option" statement was made orally, compliance was again 100% as everyone of the 109 clients asked signed the form. However, in one of the two clinics where both statements were read, compliance among 259 clients dropped to 41%, and in the other clinic compliance among 104 clients dropped to 20%. The other variable that probably accounts for the difference between the two clinics is that in the 41%-compliance clinic the statement was read by a clerk, whereas in the 20%-compliance clinic it was presented by a clinician. It is likely that the personal assurance of the person who will actually be delivering the services that refusal to sign will not affect the clients is more credible than this same statement from a nonclinician. The concerns expressed by the clients who did not sign included the effect that forwarding the information would have on future employment and loss of custody of their children, as well as fears of the information being used against them sometime in the future for some governmental purpose.

Professor Alan Westin concluded from this study that "millions of persons who are clients of government health services *do* care about the circulation of their personal data, and that their consent would *not* be freely obtained for many inadequately protected government data systems if clients really had adequate notice of what was to be done and felt they had a real choice of whether to consent or not."[21]

The results of other studies are consistent with this finding. Even in a case in which the government alleged it would only use the information contained in worker health records for the protection of the workers themselves, for example, a majority of du Pont workers refused to give OSHA access to their medical records.[22]

RELEASE FORMS

The Congressional Privacy Commission found that in many instances, when an individual applies for a job, life or health insurance, credit, or financial assistance or services from the government, he is asked to relinquish certain medical information. While believing that this was necessary in many cases, the commission also found that individuals are generally asked to sign open-ended or blanket authorizations with wording such as that requiring the recipient to "furnish any and all information on request."[23]

The American Psychiatric Association takes the position that such blanket consents are unacceptable, since they do not afford the patient the general "informed consent" protections.[24] The APA is correct. However, the commission thought the APA impractical because patients do not know precisely what information is to be disclosed or what use is likely to be made of it. Recognizing these limits, the commission made the following recommendations:

That whenever an individual's authorization is required before a medical-care provider may disclose information it collects or maintains about him, the medical-care provider should not accept as valid any authorization which is not:

(a) in writing;

(b) signed by the individual on a date specified or by someone authorized in fact to act in his behalf;

(c) clear as to the fact that the medical-care provider is among those either specifically named or generally designated by the individual as being authorized to disclose information about him;

(d) specific as to the nature of the information the individual is authorizing to be disclosed;

(e) specific as to the institutions or other persons to whom the individual is authorizing information to be disclosed;

(f) specific as to the purpose(s) for which the information may be used by any of the parties named in (e) both at the time of the disclosure and at any time in the future;

(g) specific as to its expiration date, which should be for a reasonable time not to exceed one year . . . .

Computer centers have the right to refuse to honor requests that are not specific, on the grounds that the patient probably did not understand to what he was consenting. A center should contact the patient directly if it is suspicious of the quality of the consent and thus the legality of the release form.

The commission also takes the position that when a minor is permitted to consent to treatment for specific conditions, confidentiality must be protected, and only the minor should be allowed to consent to release of medical information.

DISCLOSURE TO OTHER HEALTH PROVIDERS

Health professionals who are directly involved in the patient's care may discuss the patient's case among themselves without breaching confidentiality. However, health professionals involved in the patient's care may not discuss the patient or his case with other professionals who are not directly involved in the patient's care without the patient's consent unless the patient's identity is protected. The practical reality is that confidentiality is frequently breached in this manner, usually without the patient ever knowing of it. Physicians and other health-care professionals commonly discuss cases with other professionals, sometimes under the pretext of informal consultation, and sometimes for no better reason than that the information is somehow interesting or even titillating.

The question of access to personally identifiable medical information by members of a hospital staff or other employees needs much more attention than it has received to date. Computer centers need a clear policy on this matter.

DISCLOSURE TO FAMILY MEMBERS

While the American Medical Association contends that "reporting to one spouse information about the medical condition of the other is not a breach of confidentiality,"[25] only two cases have been found that support this proposition, and each is of dubious value. The first is a 1963 Louisiana case that rested on the proposition that the husband had a right to know about his wife's condition because "he is head and master of the family and responsible for its debts."[26] The only other case is a 1966 memorandum opinion of the New York Supreme Court sitting in Nassau County. This case also involved disclosure to a husband, and the court cited the Louisiana case in denying liability. As if unsure of his position, however, Judge Paul J. Widlitz added: "At any rate, a physician who reveals the nature of the condition of the patient to the patient's husband may hardly be charged with reprehensible conduct."[27] The better rule is that no disclosures to spouses or relatives should be permitted without the patient's express consent, and computer centers should adopt this rule.

OWNERSHIP OF MEDICAL RECORDS

The general rule is that owner of the paper on which the medical record is written is the "owner" of the record. Some states even have statutes that specify that hospitals "own" the medical records in their custody. Likewise, physicians, even if not covered by statute, can properly be considered the owners of the medical records generated and maintained by them in their private offices, and the owner of the computer data base is the "owner" of the medical records on it.

Ownership of a medical record, however, is a limited, not an absolute right, and should be considered primarily custodial in nature. Possession of the record is governed by many other statutes (e.g., state licensing statutes) and contracts (e.g., Blue Shield contracts) as well as by the interests of the patient himself in the contents of the medical record. While providers have custody of records and strong interests in them, others may have interests strong enough to give them a right of access to the information or a right to a copy of the records themselves.

PATIENT ACCESS TO MEDICAL RECORDS

In the past decade there has been a trend toward increasing patient access to medical records. This trend includes physician and hospital policy changes, judicial decisions, and state statutes and regulations, as access is generally a matter of state law.

In every state patients can obtain their records by filing a suit against the provider, usually alleging negligence, and subpoena the records for use in developing the case. In at least nine states[28] the patient is given the statutory right to inspect his hospital record without any resort to litigation. In some the statute applies only after discharge, whereas in others no such distinction is made. Statutes in some other states also have limitations on psychiatric records. In Colorado, for example, psychiatric records need not be disclosed if, in the opinion of an independent third-party psychiatrist, such disclosure to the patient "would have significant negative psychological impact upon the patient." Other states limit the types of records that are available. For example, in Minnesota access to "laboratory reports, X-rays, prescriptions, and other technical information used in assessing the patient's health condition" is specifically excluded.[29] In still others, such as Tennessee and Mississippi, the patient must show "good cause" before he has a right to view the record, but the rulings do not define what is meant by this term.[30]

Instead of requiring access to the records themselves, Florida law requires only that "reports" made of physical and mental examinations and treatments be made available to the patient.[31] Many other states have more limited statutes that either provide for access under certain circumstances, or require the patient to obtain access through an attorney, physician, or relative.[32]

Access is guaranteed by judicial decisions in other states, such as Illinois, Nebraska, New York and Texas. The general theory of the case law is that "the fiducial [trust] qualities of the physician–patient relationship require the disclosure of medical data to a patient or his agent on request . . .";[33] and that patients have a right to access to their own records based on a "Common law right of inspection."[34]

State medical licensing boards are also beginning to take cognizance of the importance of patient access to medical records. New York in 1977 and Massachusetts in 1978 have required their licensees to make such records available to patients upon request.[35] On the federal level (e.g., Veteran's Administration facilities) the Privacy Act of 1974 requires direct access under most circumstances, and the Privacy Protection Study Commission, established by that act, has recommended that:

> Upon request, an individual who is the subject of a medical record maintained by a medical-care provider, or another responsible person designated by the individual, be allowed access to that medical record including an opportunity to see and copy it.

This recommendation[36] is significantly broader than one made more than five years previously by HEW's Medical Malpractice Commission, which recommended that "states enact legislation enabling patients to obtain access to the information contained in their medical records through their legal representatives, public or private, without having to file a suit."[37] Computer centers should have a clear policy aimed at providing patients access to their own medical records in as uncomplicated a manner as possible.

IS ACCESS HARMFUL TO PATIENTS?

The argument that an ignorant patient is a happy patient is unpersuasive — especially when the patient wants specific facts. Patients who *ask* to see their own medical records are not "less anxious" when refused than they would be if access were provided. In fact, every study that has been done supports the conclusion that patient access to medical records is a positive step for patients and possesses no threat to their health care.

In one study in Burlington, Vermont, for example, staff physicians in the Rehabilitation Medicine Service at the Medical Center Hospital of Vermont routinely gave patients copies of their records. Of 103 patients surveyed, 88% registered moderate to enthusiastic interest in their medical records, 60% asked for clarification, and 50% made minor corrections in their records.[38]

An Australian study provided open access to records for hospital inpatients. Although some believed before the study that this setting "might worsen anxiety," this concern was not borne out, and the results indicated positive patient acceptance.[39] The primary problems patients had with the records involved medical abbreviations, vocabulary, and physician handwriting. The study also had some therapeutic payoffs. In two cases patients with chronic debilitating diseases expressed their unfounded fear that they had cancer only after reviewing their records, thus providing an opportunity for the physician to discuss this belief with them. In another case a pregnant woman found a mistake in her blood type where in fact an Rh incompatibility existed. Similar positive results were reported from a study in a psychiatric unit at a general hospital in the state of Washington, where inpatients were permitted to read their records at will at a central nursing station on the ward.[40] In another study at the Given Health Care Center in Burlington, Vermont, 8,000 patients were given a carbon copy of their complete office records. Ninety-three percent felt that the process reduced their anxieties about their health.[41]

Moreover, in places where access is available, no adverse reactions have been reported. In Massachusetts, for example, patient access has been generally available in hospitals since 1975 without reported incident. And the Privacy Study Commission, hearing from all federal agencies that had adopted access policies under the Privacy Act of 1974 found that "Not one witness was able to identify an instance where access to records has had an untoward effect on a patient's medical condition." Finally, a two-year study at the outpatient department of Boston's Beth Israel Hospital concluded that not only did physician fears not materialize from liberal patient access to records, but also the access policy made the relationship between patients and professionals "more collaborative."[42]

Some physicians have suggested giving all patients a carbon copy of their record as soon as it is made. The advantages of this system would include: (1) increased patient information and education; (2) continuity of records as patients move or change physicians; (3) an added criterion on which patients may base physician selection; (4) improvement in the doctor-patient relationship by making it more open; (5) an added way for physicians to monitor quality of care; and (6) increased responsiveness to consumer needs.[43] The analogue in a computerized system is open for patient access to the data about themselves in the system.

FORBIDDING ACCESS

If the patient has a statutory right to the record, there is nothing that can legally prevent the patient's access. However, inherent in the law is the notion of reasonableness. It may be reasonable for a data center to suggest that the patient's physician be present while the patient inspects the record. On the other hand, it is unreasonable to require this in most circumstances. For instance, it is unreasonable for a data center to deny the patient access to records if the patient must make a treatment decision and needs the information to do so.

Some statutes provide, and common sense dictates, that if the physician has good reason to believe that access to the record will be harmful to the patient, the access may be denied. But this provision is not to be treated casually — the physician must be reasonable in his belief, and should be able to document his belief on the basis of objective evidence. The patient should also be given the opportunity to challenge this decision, or to designate another person to receive the information for him. Data centers could develop policies consistent with the rule of reasonableness.

CORRECTING ERRORS

One of the few legal lessons most health professionals have learned is: *Never alter a medical record.* This is excellent advice, since a jury will often consider altering a medical record as the equivalent of admitting negligence. Nevertheless, like almost every rule this one has some obvious exceptions — the most obvious occurring when the record is incorrect. There have been many suggestions concerning record alteration. Perhaps the most widely recommended one is to cross out the incorrect information in such a way that it is still legible, write in the correct information, and add a dated note explaining why the information was changed (e.g., changed because it was later discovered to be inaccurate).[45] Such a procedure would both maintain the integrity of the medical record and permit the correction of false data. Each physician and hospital should have a procedure for making record corrections. In the event that the health-care provider determines that no correction is warranted, the patient should at least be permitted to have his own version of the facts added to the record. Computerized systems will have to develop rules for making changes consistent with these general guidelines.

PROVIDER PRIVACY

The question of provider privacy generally arises when a state agency demands certain information from physicians about their patients, and the physicians refuse arguing that disclosure of the information would be harmful to their patients and disrupt their practicing their profession as they deem appropriate, and therefore violate the physician's "right of privacy" implicit in the doctor-patient relationship.

This issue was raised, for example, in a challenge to a New York statute requiring that all prescriptions for schedule II drugs be made out in triplicate and that one copy be forwarded to a state agency for placement on a computer tape.[46] The physicians alleged that the statute impaired their right to practice medicine free of "unwarranted state interference" because it deterred them from writing certain prescriptions for fear their patients' records might become public. The court summarily dismissed this argument, saying that whatever right of privacy physicians had in the doctor-patient relationship was "derivative from, and therefore no stronger than, the patients'." The statute itself was upheld on the basis that it served a rational state purpose (making sure dangerous drugs were used only for legitimate medical purposes), and had sufficient built-in safeguards protecting the patient's right to privacy. Specifically, the forms were received by the state agency and coded, and the information was placed on computer tapes. The forms were put in a vault, stored for five years, and then destroyed. The room in which the tapes were kept was surrounded by a locked wire fence and protected by an alarm system. The tapes were kept in a locked cabinet, and when used, the computer was run "off-line" (i.e., no terminal outside the computer room could read or record any information). Disclosure of data was prohibited by statute and was a crime punishable by up to a year in prison. Only 17 state employees and 24 investigators were authorized to use the files.

In a related case, the Alaska Supreme Court ruled that a public official need not divulge, under their conflict of interest statutes, the names of his patients who have paid him more than $100 (at least until the state adopts provisions to protect the confidential nature of the information).[47] The court indicated that the protections should be like those in the New York drug statute. The court permitted the physician to argue that such a disclosure would violate the rights of his patients, and noted that generally the fact that a patient has gone to a particular physician is not private. However, the court thought it could be if, for example, the professional was "a psychiatrist, psychologist, or physician who specialized in treating sexual problems or venereal disease."

Experience with PSROs in the United States has indicated that providers may be more unwilling than patients to see medical records computerized because of their own concerns with how aggregate data on their own patients may be used to evaluate them as providers.

RECOMMENDATIONS OF THE PRIVACY COMMISSION

The Privacy Protection Study Commission, which was set up by Congress in 1974 to study individual privacy rights and record-keeping practices, issued its final report in July 1977. The commission based its recommendations on findings that: medical records now contain more information and are available to more users than ever before; the control of health-care providers over these records has been greatly diluted; restoration of this control is not possible; free patient consent to disclosure is generally illusory; access of patients to their records is rare; and there are steps that can be taken to improve the quality of records, enhance patient awareness of their content, and control their disclosure. Some of the commission's major recommendations are:

—that each State enact a statute creating individual rights of access to, and correction of medical records, and an enforceable expectation of confidentiality for medical records

—that federal and state penal codes be amended to make it a criminal offense for any individual knowingly to request or obtain medical record information from a medical care provider under false pretenses or through deception

—that upon request, an individual who is the subject of a medical record maintained by a medical care provider, or another responsible person designated by the individual, be allowed to have access to that medical record, including the opportunity to see and copy it; and have the opportunity to correct or amend the record

—each medical care provider be required to take affirmative measures to assure that the medical records it maintains are made available only to authorized recipients and on a "need-to-know" basis

—that any disclosure of medical-record information by a medical-care provider be limited only to information necessary to accomplish the purpose for which the disclosure is made

—that each medical care provider be required to notify an individual on whom it maintains a medical record of the disclosures that may be made of information in the record without the individual's express authorization.

SUMMARY

The recommendations of Alan Westin following his study of computerized medical records (*Computers, Health Records, and Citizen Rights,* 1976) provide a useful summary and conclusion to this chapter. In brief, he recommended public notice of all data systems; a limit on the type of personal health data collected, requiring specific release forms; easy patient access to all data about themselves; a duty to ensure accuracy, take appropriate security measures, and respect human rights on the part of the data center; independent review and public oversight of the data center; and guidelines for the use of aggregate data in research.

It is too soon to write the definitive handbook on protecting privacy in computerized medical data systems. Suffice it to say here that the issues are well outlined in the law dealing with manual records, and the principles developed there should be applied insofar as possible to computerized systems as well.

NOTES

1. Ervin, *Civilized Man's Most Valued Right,* 2 Prism 15 (June 1974); cf. A. Westin and M. Baher, *Data Banks in a Free Society* (New York: Quadrangle, 1973), pp. 17-20; A. Miller, *The Assault on Privacy* (New York: New American Library, 1972), pp. 184-220.
2. Hammonds v. Aetna Cas. & Sur. Co., 243 F. Supp. 793 (N.D. Ohio 1965).
3. In Curry v. Corn, 227 N.Y.S.2d 470 (1966), for example, the physician disclosed information to his patient's husband, who was contemplating a divorce action. In Schaffer v. Spicer, 215 N.W.2d 134 (S.D. 1974), the wife's psychiatrist disclosed information to the husband's attorney to aid him in a child custody case. Representative of the insurance cases are Hague v. Williams, 181 A.2d (N.J. 1962), where the pediatrician of an infant informed a life insurance company of a congenital heart defect that he had not informed the child's parents of, and Hammonds v. Aetna, *supra* note 2, where the physician revealed information to an insurance company when the insurance company falsely represented to him that his patient was suing him for malpractice. Cases involving reporting to employers include Beatty v. Baston, 13 Ohio L. Abs. 481 (Ohio App. 1932), where the physician revealed to a patient's employer during a workman's compensation action that the patient had venereal disease; Clark v. Geraci, 208 N.Y.S.2d 564 (S. Ct. N.Y. 1960), where a civilian employee of the Air Force asked his doctor to make an incomplete disclosure to his employer to explain absences, but the doctor made a complete disclosure including the patient's alcoholism; and the more recent case of Horne v. Patton, 287 So.2d 824 (Ala. 1973), which involved the disclosure of information not specified in the opinion.
4. 8 Wigmore on Evidence§2380a. Retention of the privilege was also the most controversial item in the new Federal Rules of Evidence. While initial versions eliminated the privilege entirely, the final version provides that the privilege shall "be governed by the principles of the common law as they may be interpreted by the courts of the United States in the light of reason and experience." Where, however, state law governs a case, the privilege shall be "determined in accordance with state law." Rule 501. There are, however, numerous exceptions to the privilege rule. The most important are:

    1. Communications made to a doctor when no doctor-patient relationship exists.
    2. Communications made to a doctor that are not for the purposes of diagnosis and treatment or are not necessary to the purposes of diagnosis and treatment (e.g., who inflicted the gunshot wound and why).
    3. In actions involving commitment proceedings, issues as to wills, actions on insurance policies.

4. In actions in which the patient brings his physical or mental condition into question (e.g., personal injury suit for damages, raising an insanity defense, malpractice action against a doctor or hospital).
5. Reports required by state statutes (e.g., gunshot wounds, acute poisoning, child abuse, motor vehicle accidents, and, in some states, venereal disease).
6. Information given to the doctor in the presence of another not related professionally to the doctor or known by the patient.

5. A. Westin, *Privacy and Freedom* (New York: Atheneum, 1967), p. 7.
6. Horne v. Patton, 287 So.2d 824 (Ala. 1973).
7. Miller, *Personal Privacy in the Computer Age,* 67 MICH. L. REV. 1089, 1107 (1968).
8. In 1939, for example, *Time* magazine published a story in its "medicine" section with a photograph of the patient, a young woman who was receiving treatment for uncontrollable gluttony apparently induced by a condition of the pancreas, Barber v. Time, Inc., 159 S.W.2d 291 (Mo. 1942). Other cases, like Horne v. Patton, *supra* note 6, however, indicate that publication is not necessary to sustain an invasion of privacy action. For example, having unauthorized persons in a delivery room, DeMay v. Roberts, 9 N.W. 146 (Mich. 1881), or, by analogy, permitting unauthorized persons to view confidential medical records, may also be an invasion of privacy.
9. California Health and Safety Code, sec. 2554 (Supp. 1970).
10. Landeros v. Flood, 17 CAL. 3d 399, 131 C 21 RPTE, 551 P2d 389 (1976).
11. N.Y. Penal Code, sec. 265.25 (Supp. 1969). And see, generally, Rose, Pathology Reports and Autopsy Protocols: Confidentiality, Privilege and Accessibility, 57 Am. J. Crim. Pro. A.J.C.P.144 (1972), and Denver Pub. Co. v. Dreyfus, 520 P.2d 104 (Col. 1974) (autopsy reports open to public under Open Records Act). A physician does not need a statute to release confidential medical information while a danger to the public exists. The leading case enunciating this exception, Simonsen v. Swenson, 177 S.W. 831, was decided by the Supreme Court of Nebraska in 1920. In that case a man who was visiting a small town was seen by a physician who was also the physician for the hotel in which the visitor was staying. The physician diagnosed syphilis and advised the patient to "get out of town" or he would tell the hotel management. When the patient remained in town, the doctor notified the landlady, who disinfected the man's room and removed his belongings to the hallway. The court decided that the doctor had the right to reveal just as much information concerning a contagious disease as was necessary for others to take proper precautions against becoming infected with it, and that his actions under the circumstances were justified.
12. Hoffman v. Blackmon, 241 So.2d 752 (Fla. App. 1970); and see Wojcik v. Aluminum Co. of America, 183 N.Y.S. 2d 351, 357-358 (1959).

13. Jones v. Stanko, 118 Ohio St. 147, 160 N.E. 456 (1928).
14. Davis v. Rodman, 147 Ark. 385, 227 S.W. 612 (1921).
15. Skillings v. Allen, 143 Minn. 323, 173 N.W. 663 (1919).
16. Tarasoff v. Regents of U. of California, 131 Cal. Rpt. 14, 551 P.2d 334 (1976).
17. See A. Stone, The Tarasoff Decisions: Suing Psychotherapists to Safeguard Society, 90 Harv. L. Rev. 358 (1976).
18. Under a similar theory, clauses by which the patient has agreed not to sue the hospital for negligence have been ruled invalid because the patient really had no choice but to sign the form. Tunkl v. Regents of Univ. of California, 60 Cal.2d 92, 383 P.2d 441 (1963). One could argue that it is impossible to give consent for release of medical records before they are in existence (e.g., at the beginning of a hospital stay rather than at the end), since at that time one may have no reasonable idea of what they might contain.
19. Note, *Medical Practice and the Right to Privacy,* 43 MINN. L. REV. 943, 960 (1959).
20. This study, called "The Georgia 'Free Consent' Experiment," is described in A. Westin, *Computers, Health Records, and Citizen Rights,* National Bureau of Standards Monograph 157 (Washington, D.C.: U.S. Gov. Printing Office, 1976), at 243-245.
21. *Id.* at 245.
22. *Id.*
23. *Personal Privacy in an Information Society* (Washington, D.C.: U.S. Gov. Printing Office, 1977).
24. *Id.* citing A.P.A., Confidentiality and Third Parties, APA; Washington, D.C., 1975 at 13.
25. *Disclosure of Confidential Information,* 216 JAMA 385 (1971).
26. Pennison v. Provident Life & Accident Ins. Co., 154 So.2d 617, 618 (La. Ct. App., 1963).
27. Curry v. Corn, 217 N.Y. S.2d 470, 472, 52 Misc. 2d 1035 (1966).
28. Colorado (Col. Rev. Stat. § 25-1-801), Oklahoma (Okla. Stat. Ann. 76 § 19), Connecticut (Conn. Gen. Stat. Ann. § 4.104), Illinois (Ill. St. 51 § 71), Indiana (Ind. St. 34-3-15.5-4), Nevada (Nev. R.S. 629.061), Massachusetts (Mass. G. L. ch. 111, § 70), New York (N.Y. ch. 44, § 17), Pennsylvania (Pa. St. 51 § 71).
29. Minn. 144.335(2) (amended, 1976).
30. Tenn. 53-1322 (1974); Miss. § 41-9-65 (1962).
31. Fla. Stat. Ann. § 458.16.
32. For example, Maine, Missouri, Montana, New Jersey, New Mexico, North Dakota, Utah, Wisconsin, Hawaii, California. For a state-by-state breakdown and description of specific statutory provisions see M. Auerback, and T. Bogue, *Getting Yours: A Consumer Guide to Obtaining Your Medical*

Record (1978), Health Research Group, 2000 P St., Washington, D.C. 20036 ($2).
33. Cannell v. Medical and Surgical Clinic, 315 N.E. 2d 278, 280 (Ill. App. Ct. 3d Dist. 1974).
34. Hutchins v. Texas Rehabilitation Comm., 544 S.W. 2d 802, 804 (Tex. Ct. Civ. App. 1976). *See also,* O'Donnell v. Sherman, Sup. Ct., Middlesex No. 77-4622 (Mass., May 22, 1978, Doerfer, J.). *Contra,* Gotkin v. Miller, 379 F. Supp. 815, (N.Y. 1978) *aff'd,* 514 F.2d 123 (2d Cir. 1975) (former mental patient does not have a constitutional right to a copy of her records under New York law). See, generally, B. Kaiser, *Patient's Right of Access to Their Own Medical Records: The Need for New Law.*
35. The full regulation, which was adopted on October 10, 1978, reads:

REQUIREMENT TO MAKE AVAILABLE CERTAIN RECORDS

a. A licensee shall maintain a medical record for each patient which is adequate to enable the licensee to provide proper diagnosis and treatment. A licensee must maintain a patient's medical record for a minimum period of three years from the date of the last patient encounter and in a manner which permits the former patient or a successor physician access to them in conformity with this section.

b. A licensee shall provide a patient or, upon a patient's request, another licensee or another specifically authorized person, with the following:
   i. A summary, which includes all relevant data, of that portion of the patient's medical record which is in the licensee's possession, or a copy of that portion of the patient's entire medical record which is in the licensee's possession. It is within the licensee's discretion to determine whether to make available a summary or a copy of the entire medical record.
   ii. A copy of any previously completed report required for third party reimbursement.

c. A licensee may charge a reasonable fee for the expense of providing the material enumerated in section b.; however, a licensee may not require prior payment of the charges for the medical services to which such material relates as a condition for making it available.

d. Section b. does not apply if, in the reasonable exercise of her professional judgment, a licensee believes the provision of such material would adversely affect the patient's health. However, in such a case, the licensee must make the material available to another responsible person designated by the patient. 243 CMR 2.06 (13).

36. *Secretary's Report on Medical Malpractice,* HEW, DHEW Pub. No. OS 73-88,1973 at 77.

37. A. Golodetz, J. Ruess, and R. Milhous, *The Right to Know: Giving the Patient his Medical Record,* 57 Arch. Phys. Med. Rehab. 78 (1976).

38. D. Stevens, R. Stagg, and I. MacKay, *What Happens When Hospitalized Patients See Their Own Records,* 86 Ann. Intern. Med. 474 (1977).

39. E. Stein, et al., *Patient Access to Medical Records on a Psychiatric Inpatient Unit* 136 Am. J. Psychiatry 3 (1979).

40. R. Bouchard et al., reported in "How to Reduce Patients' Anxiety: Show Them Their Hospital Records," *Medical World News,* Jan. 13, 1975, at 48.

41. R. Knox, "Medical board told patients should get access to records," *Boston Globe,* March 2, 1978, at 15.

42. Shenkin and Warner, *Giving the Patient His Medical Record: A Proposal to Improve the System,* 289 New Eng. J. Med. 688 (1973). See also, Letters to the Editor in response to the proposal, 290 New Eng. J. Med. 287-288 (1974).

43. Rabens v. Jackson Park Hosp. Foundation, 351 N.E. 2d 276 (Ill. 1976).

44. *See, e.g.,* S. Babin, *Changing Notes in Medical Records: A Proposal,* 6(1) Medicolegal News 4 (Spring 1978).

45. Whalen v. Roe, 429 U.S. 589 (1977).

46. Falcon v. Alaska Public Offices Com'n., 570 P.2d 469 (Alaska 1977).

6
COMPUTERS IN HOSPITALS

Donald Fenna, Ph.D.
The University of Alberta Edmonton,
Alberta, Canada

As larger elements of the health care delivery system, hospitals have been natural foci for implementation of the capital-intensive computer. In the 1960s the high cost of even a modest computer and poor facilities for sharing, restricted computer use to large institutions. The development of time-sharing systems in the late 1960s and early 1970s removed one impediment to use, and allowed a pay-for-what-you-need approach. Concurrent development of the minicomputer, then of the microcomputer, opened the door to widespread use. Size is no longer important re hardware; any size hospital can have one, and computers may be numerous within a single hospital. However, while obviating conflict in the sharing of a single computer, and allowing ready acquisition of specialty systems, this trend has often had negative aspects. Too often, the computers serve in disparate rather than coordinated ways. It is common for laboratories and radiology to duplicate the work of the admitting office. It is common for clinical and business elements of an institution to enter the same data separately. But, while smallness and cheapness are facilitating proliferation and thus encouraging competition rather than cooperation, other forces, including growing experience, tend to oppose this. Current trends are toward thorough and comprehensive integration within the hospital, and toward integration across ambulatory care and family practice too.

THE BUSINESS OFFICE

Though incidental to the care of the patient, the business office has been the pioneer focus of computer application in most hospitals. This applies particularly in the United States, where income is not only tied to service rendered but may be dictated by the individual item of service. The amount of data required by the U. S. business office is immense compared, for instance, with that in Canada or Europe, where most inpatient care is free, and any charges are on an inclusive per diem basis.

Several factors favored this line of entry of the computer into the hospital, apart from volume of data. One such factor was the relative simplicity of assessing benefits of improved processing; whether it was the capturing of more items or more prompt capturing (particularly in the context of impending discharge), a dollar figure was easily established. Second, accounts receivable, payroll, and general ledger were applications common to other industries that had automated; although usually more complicated in hospitals, the methodologies of more innovative industries could be followed. Further, it has usually been easier for business-office-sponsored computer proposals to be funded for nonpragmatic management needs. In addition, medical insurance organizations have often helped explore computerization of financial procedures for associated hospitals — overtly to aid cost containment but also because of the growth aspirations of insurers.

Foremost among the differences between accounting in hospitals and other industries is the matter of insurance coverage. In most countries that levy a service charge to the patient for hospitalization there are schemes of insurance to cover prospective patients. There are often parallel schemes serving people of different socioeconomic status, and competing schemes for any one client or group of clients. And there are often layers of insurance coverage applying to one patient. Except when the patient has to pay all the claim (and even this may require an elaborate statement from the hospital), this variety can produce a labyrinthine accounting system. Since direct billing of insurers tends to reduce bad debts and expedite processing, it is usual. Hence so is the labyrinth, with two, three, or even more parties each assigned a part of the total bill, the proportions perhaps depending on the particular scheme of coverage chosen by the patient. The computer system requires correspondingly greater investment in program development than applies to other industries, but the completed system has similarly increased payback. It is now routine for such multiple billing to be done by computer, and for the transactions between hospital and insurer to be conducted via magnetic tape or electronic communication.

The payroll is another fiscal area where hospitals tend to be more complicated than other industries. The plethora of professions in hospitals and the wide variety of types of staff compound inherent complications. Many hospitals have several unions and over a dozen labor agreements — for a staff that may number barely a few thousand. Round-the-clock operations bring shift differentials, on-call allowances, call-back pay with minimum attendance provisions, and various responsibility components into the formal agreements. Elaborate costing schemes may be required, for example, to cover "floating pool" nurses; this particular facet is particularly relevant with the trend toward dynamic variable staffing of nursing stations. Trends toward "program budgeting" and "zero-based budgeting" — prompted largely by the widespread concern over escalating costs — are adding to the demand.

PATIENT INFORMATION SYSTEM — REGISTRATION

One step toward patient care takes us from the business office to the admitting office: from the recording of a patient just as a fee-paying customer to the recording as a client of the care service. The admitting office usually acts as the front-end of the business office, but it acts quite distinctly as the front-end for medical records too. Importantly from the viewpoint of patient care, it can set up basic documents for a case history, including, in most hospitals, identification of the new admittee in the context of a central patient register.

For larger and longer-established hospitals the identification of patients relative to the central register is far from simple. Erroneous identification is not unusual. With an accumulated population of hundreds of thousands of patients, even the most diligent search of manual or mechanized files can result in a false conclusion. Add discrepancies in the patient's presented details, mistakes in comprehension, errors in previous manual filing, and stresses of the moment, and the risk of false conclusion increases considerably. The computer has brought many improvements. It is rigorous in its filing. It does not have to withdraw a record just because it is being viewed. It makes available simultaneously to its widespread users every record it has — immediately upon the creation of each. And it can maintain a variety of cross indices (e.g., by insurance number and birthdate as well as the usual name). In sophisticated developments it provides means for searching in some approximate sense, thereby avoiding many problems caused by inconsistencies of spelling and dating. A phonetic edition of the name annuls the differences between Macphee and McPhee and MacFie, and between Nelson and Nielson and Neilsen. More sophisticated systems assess the match of new and old in terms of literal surname, phonetic surname, first name, second initial, sex, birth year, birth month, and birth day — applying appropriate weights to offset mere chance. A returning patient may thus be detected despite a change of surname and the adoption of a false age. Where surnames are very common, inclusion of mother's maiden name is often added to break free of the widespread uniformity.

The early developments of computerized central registers used batch processing, which precluded any automatic searching in "real time" but at least made comprehensive directories available to multiple points. Such directories, often now on microfiche rather than paper, persist as back-up for failed real-time systems. Many early real-time systems used on-line typewriters as the entry device as well as for printing admitting forms, but, as in most fields now, the cathode ray tube has become the normal means for displaying entered data (i.e., newly entered or previously entered data furnished in response to a query). This change to a visual display terminal was crucial to the general acceptability of the application, the slowness of the typewriter being unsatisfactory in most situations. The scene in many hospitals today has each admitting officer operating a keyboard-equipped video display terminal while interviewing the patient. After entry of general identification data, a list of patients meeting the criteria is displayed. Selection of any one, or entry of an identification number in the first place, prompts display of the previously entered data on the patient. This information is then checked and amended where necessary, prior to automatic production of the admission form. This procedure will become commonplace, even in small hospitals, as computerized records become the benchmark.

The methodology for video terminals has yet to settle to one preferred style. The simpler terminals operate in a "conversational" mode, and have a normal keyboard for entry of data. More complicated terminals operate in "page mode," with a whole screenful of data moving at any time between computer and terminal; the keyboard may have many extra keys for special functions, including selection from preferred alternatives on the screen. Other terminals have a "light pen" instead of some such function keys, allowing the user to select by pointing (i.e., touching the screen location with the pen). And the simple two-tone screen may now have selective flashing, double intensity, or reverse illumination of characters. Colored screens are coming into use.

There is a need to offer alternative methodologies to users of differing familiarity. Whereas an unfamiliar user requires help at each step, with textual explanations and step-by-step progress, the fully familiar user wants the ability to enter abbreviated codes and facility to complete a transaction as a single operation, with no explanatory intrusions.

Besides its speed, the video terminal avoids unnecessary consumption of paper; all its displaying is via the transient medium of the screen. However, until such time as the whole patient record is computerized and universally accessible, a paper record will continue. This purpose is served by the admitting form, which is usually produced by a computer-driven typewriter in the admitting office, but can also be made via an in-built copying unit in the video terminal.

While it is customary for each inpatient to be given a unique lifetime identity number, it is not so common to do the same for patients of outpatient departments, and it is still less common for a hospital to assign one such number to a patient for all purposes. Physical size and spread have been major inhibitors of "unified numbering." The computer, particularly in real-time mode, bypasses such problems, and also facilitates greater interdepartmental availability of general record data. Relative to its own information, the computer introduces a unified record, although it may thus make less necessary the unification of the paper records. For the outpatient clinics it is possible to imagine operation without any formal paper record, a reception procedure similar to that of the admitting office being followed by entry of observations, orders, and so on.

Choosing the number to be used as the common unified number within the hospital has itself caused problems and soul-searching, at least in North America. In the absence of a health care identity number as found in the countries that have national socialized health systems, and the even more general identity number of some others, resort has often been made to the social security/ insurance number. However, besides its absence for most younger patients, changing attitudes in society have brought increasing opposition to the wider use of such numbers. Numbers separately assigned by each hospital are thus the norm, even in the more socialized and integrated health care system of Canada. Regional numbering schemes, encompassing several hospitals and also family practice and other private clinics, are discussed, but probably as fast as the industry interest rises, so does the opposition of a public grown skeptical and afraid of computerized data banks. Some proposals have been made for using a number encoding various characteristics of the patient, but use of a simple meaningless number is the only efficient, problem-free scheme.

With hundreds and sometimes thousands of current inpatients, keeping track of their locations is a major task in many hospitals. Hence, it is usual for any computerized inpatient registration system to include all transfer and discharge elements as well as admission (the composite system often being given the illogical title "Admission-Discharge-Transfer"). Discharges, and many transfers, are essential data for accounting on the one hand and utilization studies on the other. The current location is essential to routing the visitor, the phlebotomist and other traveling technicians, drugs and other material issues, and the reports emanating from service departments. In lesser systems, knowledge of transfers and discharges passes to the admitting office, and only then enters the computer. In more extensive systems, staff at nursing stations enter this information.

THE NURSING STATION

The inpatient nursing station is the hub of the hospital; around it circulate the patients and care staff, and through it pass virtually all of the data concerning the care of the patient. Through it passes also, indirectly but decisively, the major share of a typical hospital's budget. The nursing care payroll alone absorbs about a third of this budget. Whether salaried via the hospital or remunerated through another route, the physician costs would add considerably to this expense. It is not surprising, therefore, that computerization of the general nursing station has been a long-standing aspiration.

Many major hospital computer projects of the 1960s, rationalizing and extrapolating from the pioneer developments in the field, and focusing on the nursing station as an essential part, placed terminals at each station in the subject hospital. However, the task attempted was usually too large and more complex than expected, so that the timetable was necessarily more protracted than anticipated. So, although various projects from that time or later have borne fruit in this domain, the 1980s have begun with terminals on an inpatient station as very much the exception.

Various assessment studies have indicated that 20 to 25% of a nurse's time is spent on clerical work; so both functionally and economically there is considerable potential return for computerization. Much of this work relates to medical orders that must pass to laboratories and other separate servicing units, or to the responses from such; for both of these needs the computer terminal at the station can greatly expedite action and reaction, adding further to the return on investment. Through knowledge of medication orders and so on, the computer can readily prepare medication and other schedules, facilitating accurate work within a shift and the transfer of responsibilities from shift to shift. Where patient classification (in terms of care level) and variable staffing are practiced, like expedition applies to the communication with nursing administration (and the calculation of classification from observed parameters), allowing more responsiveness in staffing. Then what have been the impediments?

The impediments have been many. For one, the equipment required for such a disseminated real-time system requires a considerable new financial commitment, for terminals and for associated central equipment. This impediment is a progressively reducing one because of the continuing cost reductions that derive from advancing electronic technology. Second, the system requirements are vastly more complex than first presumed, adding to the time scale for development and investment required, and to the hardware requirements. Third, while most hospitals use preprinted forms for many orders, overall standardization is not so usual, and in many activities procedures, styles, and expressions are highly individual, handicapping both the development of a common system and its implementation. Fourth, the fact that so much of a nurse's time is spent on clerical activities is no indicator of the aptitude for and attitude toward a computer terminal of any nurse. Nurses are typically not machine-oriented, not even typewriter-oriented; so it cannot be presumed that they will readily accept and use a computer terminal. Prior to the computer it had become common to employ ward clerks to lift some clerical load from the nurses, and in many computer developments this pattern of work disposition has been extended so that a clerk rather than a nurse handles the terminal. However, while avoiding the personality incompatibility and ostensibly putting a lower-cost employee at the keyboard, the interposition of the clerk necessitates a written instruction from the nurse, thereby negating the gain.

This design conflict, which applies at least as strongly relative to routine use of a terminal by a physician, has prompted various experimentation with terminals. One of the earliest terminals tried on a nursing station used an array of 20 X 10 labeled buttons, by which the nurse's choice was expressed. Since 200 choices wouldn't cover all laboratory tests or all drugs, a set of different overlays was provided, to be chosen among as the first step. In at least one major project, this was augmented by a second such machine, since choosing a drug, for instance, had to be accompanied by other choices (e.g., strength, frequency). Such machines avoided use, or even sight, of a keyboard for these predefined purposes, but could not cover all entry needs (e.g., an amorphous comment). Nor could they display any information that the computer could give. So they were joined by at least a keyboard and a printer or videoscreen, and in reality by a printer and a videoscreen, plus one or even two associated keyboards. This physically large array of equipment becomes inhibiting in itself, as well as both expensive and demanding of space. Subsequent developments included touch-sensitive screens with back-projected color-slides showing alternatives, then the present culmination of a light-pen-equipped video terminal. The usual requirement for a paper record of much information still demands the printer, but this too is becoming more adaptable, by a reduction in noise level for impact printers but even more so with the copier embedded in the video terminal. Another technological development that has facilitated the accommodation of terminals on crowded nursing stations, somewhat at odds with the light pen and the embedded printer, has been the separation of keyboard and screen. This allows the bulky screen to adorn a wall rather than the desk.

Two general trends with video terminal technology that have improved usability everywhere are the more capacious screen and the embedding of microprocessors to create the "intelligent terminal." (The cost of such an enhanced terminal is the same as that of its primitive predecessor of ten or more years ago.)

INTERACTING SUB-SYSTEMS — THE LABORATORY AND RADIOLOGY

With its high volume of formalized business and strong emphasis on numerical data, the laboratory was one of the initial targets in the application of the computer to clinical data. In the 1960s (and earlier), there was even a distinct computational load in the laboratory as analogue records from simple automatic analyzers were read, corrected for drift, and converted to clinical values. The large volume of business in many laboratories, plus the considerable annual growth in volume that was (and still is) occurring, also prompted demand for processing relative to business statistics for use in management decision-making.

The approaches adopted were quite varied, ranging from the direct attachment of analyzers to computers through provision of standard teletypewriters in the laboratories to traditional recording followed by punching into cards. As with all data processing, the earlier the capture of the data by machine the better, generally. Hence the first approach had to be seen as the most profitable in the long run, and the last the least. The first was, of course, also the most problematical, and the last the least. Direct attachment has in time become much easier, with the progressive displacement of the simple automatic analyzers by ones that give digital output (and in later years by the development of analyzers that embed microprocessors).

The advanced computer system installed in a laboratory today is derived from the bolder of those beginnings, and includes direct attachment of all the considerable array of automatic analyzers, plus compact specialized terminals alongside the other analyzers. Figure 1 shows such a scene.

Following entry of the test requests, the system produces collection lists for the phlebotomists. For these to be practical and efficient the computer must know both location of each patient and the geographical relationship of all the locations. The latter requires a reference file that is updated only when locations are added or altered, or the preferred routing is changed. Each patient location can be entered as part of the request, but it is usual to have a standing file on each known patient, and desirable to have this file updated as regards location independently of the test requests.

After the collection rounds, the computerized record is updated, usually on an exception basis, to reflect failures to collect, and specimen numbers are established. The computer then proceeds to prepare work lists for the various work stations in the laboratory department, again using a reference file to relate need to action. For automated equipment using multispecimen trays or the equivalent, the work lists specify the sequences of specimens, including interleaved controls and standards.

The on-line connection of automatic analyzer and computer allows the results to enter the latter without human intervention. However, it is not usually deemed desirable for results to pass unseen; usually the computer displays its garnered values for perusal by the pertinent technician, with verification entered by a simple action unless changes are seen as necessary. Besides any conversion, or connection for base-line drift, that may be required for the analyzer, the computer can compare the derived values with defined or observed norms prior to the display for the technician, highlighting any questionable results.

For manually executed tests the technician enters the concluded result via an ordering typewriter terminal or keyboard-equipped video terminal. Where the test involves counting, including differential counting, by the technician, a modified terminal may act as both counter and results conveyor. For most biochemistry and hematology tests the physical size of the full alphanumeric keyboard can be an embarrassing intruder at the bench, as can the larger style of video screen, so a specialized terminal merits consideration just on physical grounds.

Once known and verified in the computer, the results may be printed there for distribution or made available to remote terminals. Most existing laboratory systems offer the alternatives, but few implement the more expeditious latter

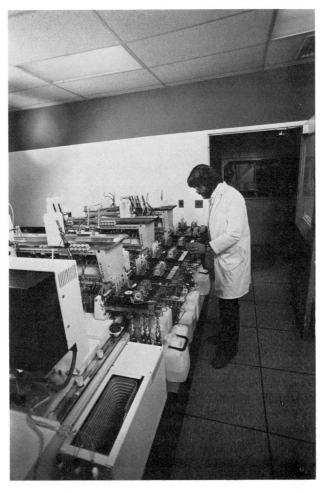

Figure 1. Prisma. AutoChemistry Department. Machine has ability to process multiple chemistry tests rapidly and accurately. (Courtesy MetPath, New Jersey.)

alternative generally. Unless a comprehensive hospital information system has terminals spread through the nursing stations, and is connected to the laboratory system, justification for distributed terminals will likely be limited to the more critical care units and any faraway stations. For out-of-hospital destinations, automatic or semiautomatic resort to public telegraphic services can be made.

Three stages of publication of results can be recognized — the first relating to the result of each individual test, the second to the set of results for each request, the third to the cumulative picture. While it is not generally efficient to print and distribute the partial results of stage one, the individual results can easily and efficiently be made available to the remote terminals, and the incomplete sets printed for distribution where missing elements are seen as unduly delaying the available results. All of these options apply comparably in noncomputerized systems, though not with the same smooth facility or normal expedition. The same does not hold for stage three — the cumulative report. Very few manual systems attempted to maintain any cumulative picture other than the crude one provided by the shingling of accumulating separate reports. Assuming capacity in the computer for retention of results for several days or more, the cumulative record for each patient can be printed in a coordinated manner that places all results for any one type of test together. Arranged in columnar format, this presentation can convey a degree of graphical image, as Figure 2 shows. Rejoined systems offer a true graphical picture, in the form of a line graph, a simulated graph, or a histogram.

The issuance of cumulative reports enhances appreciation of the patient's observed condition by the attending staff, and facilitates the manual analysis of records for discharge summaries or research. It also reduces the size of the physical record if the preceding lesser reports are discarded (though it adds to the paper consumed).

The clinical laboratory application has been a frequent target of "stand-alone" "turnkey" systems. The distinctive interfacing requirements in the laboratory were undoubtedly a factor in the development of stand-alone systems — interfacing that was much more difficult for the earlier analyzers. Until relatively recently, such interfacing was realistically achievable only with small computers, for few large computers offered the facilities, and few of those could be assigned to the engrossing task of developing the interconnections. Most of the early systems were in fact either commensurate only with a modest-sized laboratory or based on multicomputers in order to match the volume of a larger laboratory. One of the more successful products of the late sixties/early seventies used three minicomputers for three distinct tasks: one to receive and process into digital form the continuously varying analogue output of the single-channel autoanalyzers; one to assemble all the digital results, whether from the first computer, more advanced autoanalyzers, or keyboard entry; and one to handle the requisition in the first place and produce the reports afterward.

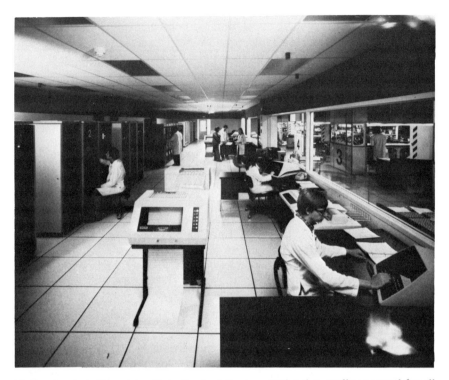

Figure 2. AutoChemistry Data Control Center. Maintains quality control for all specimens passing through AutoChemists. The AutoChemist processes the Met-Path Chem-Screen profile, a 26-chemistry-test panel. (Courtesy MetPath, New Jersey.)

The growth in power and versatility of minicomputers has removed the restraints indicated above, and even the newer microcomputers are becoming commensurate with the task. The demise of analogue output from analyzers has also facilitated interfacing, and the small microcomputers often now embedded in laboratory instruments are accentuating it. It would now be relatively easy to have the laboratory application, inclusive of its real-time on-line interaction with instruments, running merely as part of a comprehensive hospital system on a general computer. However, the considerable expertise and investment already established within specialty businesses retard any trend toward such rationalization. Moreover, despite ten or more years of background and experience, there is a dearth of well-designed laboratory systems in the marketplace. Even the most successful entrepreneurs of any particular time seem to have faded or passed away; yesterday's aggressive tenderer is often tomorrow's nonsupplier. As with so many other computer applications, particularly in hospitals, the complexity and variety of the processes and requirements are much greater than initially envisioned; so the endeavor to create a product suitable for many users is often frustrated. Despite widespread use of many common analyzers, and a generally similar approach by clinical pathologists, it remains very difficult to acquire a laboratory computer system of prior demonstrable performance and easy adaptability.

The focus of most laboratory computer systems is biochemistry and hematology, but blood banking, microbiology, and anatomic pathology are often included, and the basic reporting system is often available for other tests (e.g., electrocardiograms). Because of the need for a standing master file of current patients, many laboratory packages include an admissions component, able to support the admissions office. Many United States–based packages also include a billing component. While admirable in one sense for adding these related activities to the basic laboratory processing, such systems inherently conflict with more general hospital systems, which must include admission processes and patient registry.

The radiology department is another clinical service unit that often has a stand-alone system, for which available packages also usually include admissions and billing. Unlike pathology laboratories, radiology maintains information on past patients for a considerable time, typically a minimum of five years. This procedure, reflecting the need to keep the unwieldy X-ray film in addition to reports that can be included in any general medical record folder, has often led to radiology departments maintaining a separate patient registry from any in general use for the hospital. In some hospitals the absence of a comprehensive central register has necessitated this, while throughout North America the tendency to have radiological services provided under contract to a private practice rather than via direct employment has encouraged autonomy.

Patient bookings and registration of attendance have usually been important facets of any radiology system, in addition to the patient registry and associated identification. Control of film loans has been another facet, and preparation of reports another. Some of these applications have their parallels elsewhere in the hospital, but film control and report preparation are distinctive for radiology. In substance, film control is like control of medical record folders, but the intensity of movement distinguishes the radiology example, particularly in teaching hospitals. The basic processing for film control is not complex, and can be provided via keyboard terminals or appropriate transaction points. For high-volume situations, increasing attention is being given to automatic readers, using bar-codes or other machine-legible identification in the record covers. The same technology is being tried for the general medical record, and routine use seems to be a coming feature of physical-records control in the typical hospital.

Expeditious preparation of a verified formal report is a necessary target wherever interpretation by specialist radiologists is done. Until recently this involved dictation, transcription, and proofreading, followed by retyping whenever significant error was made; this process could easily cover two working days. Experimentation and development with computers has not only simplified the correction process but short-circuited the dictation–transcription stage. The radiologist can operate a machine that proffers alternatives for the various report contexts. The "normal" report for a given examination can be selected simply, resulting in a standard set of text. For the "abnormal," the range of alternatives offered must be extensive if the process is to be cost-effective. The menu-selection approach widely used in other computer applications, with layer after layer of alternatives appearing on the CRT screen as each simple selection is made, has been tried here. However, it is difficult to make such a laborious operation cost-effective for frequent use by a professional radiologist (and likewise for many other situations in fact). It is equally unacceptable to ask that the radiologist type in any extensive textual language. The compromise requires something more special than the ordinary CRT terminal, with a single display covering all aspects of one interpretation sentence. Such a display device, must have alternative displays if the range of radiological procedures is to be covered efficiently.

COMPUTERS FOR WORD PROCESSING

An alternative technique for facilitating the production of radiology reports is computerized word processing. While reverting to a secretarial keyboard, the ease of structuring and modifying the report in a word processor offsets the cost of dictation and transcription enough to make this newest technique competitive with the alternative discussed above. Add the weight of tradition, and it seems likely that dictation plus word processing will be the preferred means for the abnormal report, with automatic production of standard text for the normal. Currently such word processing is performed via specialty computer systems, but the future should see the embedding of word processing in the general computer system.

Most of the facilities of a word processor have been available via large computers for years; what is different today is their availability on very small computers plus cosmetic enhancements to suit a secretary. The "text editors" of the larger computers have been used for preparing various manuals for use in hospitals, including procedure manuals, general catalogs, and formularies. Initially the only form of output available was the typical inelegant computer "tab stock" report, but the 1970s have seen a burgeoning of more elegant outputs, including microfilm/microfiche, automatic phototypesetting, and the laser-beam printer. The latter two techniques automatically select bold italics or ordinary face, pack text into lines and pages, extract the table of contents, and construct the index. While automatic typesetting is undoubtedly the more elegant technique, the new laser-beam printing is much more economical, especially for larger runs.

COMPUTERS AND INSTRUMENTATION

The computer is a natural tool for analysis of data obtained by instruments, and often for controlling such instruments too. Since the normal computer functions with discrete numbers and the normal instrument produces only a continuously varying signal — i.e., the computer is "digital" and the instrument "analogue" — appropriate conversion must be made in the interface. Akin to reversing the familiar procedure of drawing a graph from a set of points or a histogram, this analogue-to-digital conversion is easily effected, but must be adequately serviced in frequency of sampling and in precision of measurement.

The minicomputers that evolved in the 1960s were sufficiently small and low in cost to allow their dedication to various instrumentation applications — the clinical laboratory with its automatic analyzers being one and the electrocardiogram another. The latter presented more problems than the former because of both its inherent greater complexity and the lack of formal scientific definition of the criteria for interpretation. The complexity constrained analysis to more powerful computers and made difficult the automatic recognition and measurement of fair sample waves. Formal definitions were developed as need arose, and various methodologies of analysis/interpretation were pursued by researchers in the field. Facilitated by the continuing improvement in power of the smaller computer, computerized measurement and interpretation of the electrocardiogram are now widespread in and outside of hospitals, and in many areas no human verification is required for "normals." However, widespread concurrence on criteria is still lacking among cardiologists, and what has long been seen as a potentially routine matter of machine processing remains largely the province of subjective art. Perhaps one reason for this is that the computer has essentially been used to imitate the cardiologist rather than gain additional insight from the waveforms — even quantitative estimates of components of the heart and its dynamics. (Some similar work on electroencephalograms is indicating diagnostic differences in the frequency spectrum that are not humanly discernible.)

The simultaneously increasing power and diminishing cost (and size) of computers are making computers more and more often an integral part of instruments, and resulting in new diagnostic or therapeutic methods entering the user market already computerized. If electrocardiography were invented only today, it would be unlikely that a noncomputerized form would ever become known. For some new methods it is doubtful that they could exist without the computer, "CT scans" being a notable example. With computerized tomography the computer not only reads and measures the rapidly changing signal but then processes mathematically a vast array of numbers before constructing an image of the biological scene. Less conspicuously, the microcomputer is becoming a standard component of various laboratory instruments, making their outputs not only digital but corrected for drift and other anomalies of the instrument and converted to ordinary clinical values. This microprocessor trend has the effect of reducing the justification for decentralized speciality computers, as mentioned earlier, pointing to a future in which one central computer is on-line to instruments while concurrently serving patient records, the business office, and so on.

A miniature of this scene exists in the confines of many intensive care units where a single computer handles nurses' notes, medication orders, and lab results while simultaneously monitoring pulse and temperature, venous and arterial pressures, weight of accumulated fluid discharged, and so on. In some such systems the computer controls the infusion of blood or nitroprusside solution within the confines of prescribed rate and amount but adjusted according to monitored pressure or fluid loss. The automatic monitoring of patients is heavily dependent on development of sensor instruments that are reliable at the necessary levels of sensitivity, and is also influenced by the ease of use of such sensors, for instance by being noninvasive. Since the computer is so diligent and so acute in its observation, and able to take heavy computations in its stride, computerized monitoring appears to be a burgeoning item in tomorrow's hospital.

THE COMPUTER, THE BEDSIDE, AND THE MEDICAL RECORD

A notable difference between hospital inpatient care and ambulatory care is that in the former the doctor normally moves among his patients, while in the latter the patients move by the doctor. Thus, while it is quite conceivable that the doctor in a clinic abjures paper records and relies entirely on a computerized record accessed via a desk-top terminal, such a paperless life lies further ahead for the hospital doctor. A terminal at a nursing station is an inadequate substitute, since it provides no means for recording or seeing information while with the patient. Unitl suitable equipment is provided at each bedside, it appears unlikely that there will be any significant reduction in the physical (paper) record. With current technology and prices, such widespread availability of computer terminals is grossly uneconomic for the general acute-care scene. However, the major development efforts aimed at providing home access to public data services could change such economics considerably over the next few years. Some form of integrated use of telephone and television will ultimately be commonplace for data purposes, and will likely revolutionize the medical record in hospitals.

RELIABILITY OF COMPUTERIZED SYSTEMS

Having developed equipment that can work for years without failure in the farthest reaches of the solar system, the electronics industry obviously can produce equipment of appropriate reliability for hospitals and other medical care. However, reliability costs money, so, like security and some other appurtenances, it is often inadequate in budget-limited developments. Virtually all computerized systems in hospitals thus suffer intermittent failure, causing direct inconvenience and a need for back-up procedures and records. The latter can erode severely the profit of computerization, while the former reduces its general acceptability. The reliability of electronics used is continually improved, but the growing permeation of computer applications increases the impact of failures. Failure of components is inevitable, but the impact can be reduced to acceptable proportions by using multiple parallel components — whether in the form of side-by-side computers or side-by-side units within a single multiprocessor computer. Equipment of the latter type is now in use in selected hospitals and will become increasingly common, its multiunit concept allowing greater flexibility in size and expansion as well as providing high reliability. Until the technology extends down to very small computers, this development must prompt a trend toward centralized rather than decentralized data storage and records processing in hospitals (the proliferation of embedded microcomputers preventing any assertion of centralized computers).

7
THE COMPUTER IN
GENERAL MEDICAL PRACTICE*

G.R. Simpson, B.A., M.B., Ch.B. (N.Z.)
Grove Clinic
Lessmurdie, W.A. Australia

INTRODUCTION

Many medical information systems discussed in papers and books are based on a number of theoretical applications[1] and have not been developed or tested in a working environment in medical practice. As a result of this lack of experience with real-life situations, they usually contain a number of theoretical applications resulting in serious errors in design that would make the system unworkable in a normal active practice.

Why has the medical profession to date not made active use of computer systems in practice, as has the rest of the business and professional community? There are three major reasons. First is the matter of cost. In most other working environments it is possible to develop data-handling techniques or introduce computer control of processes in such a way that the system becomes immediately cost-justified and in many cases profitable. Such savings are not normally available in medical practice. Second, it is not yet possible to include in an already heavily loaded medical curriculum any training in the use of computer systems, and it is therefore unusual to find a doctor who feels confident in a computer-assisted environment. Third, medical data storage and retrieval has its own peculiar requirements, and the nature of medical training and its application in practice, based as it is on a large degree of empirical information, leads to a degree of individuality in practice that creates extreme problems in designing a computer system that would be universally acceptable.

The material presented here has been developed and tested on an IBM system 32 small business computer with a 16K central core, a 9-megabyte disk storage capacity, a 100-line-per-minute printer, and a diskette drive for handling off-line

---

[†]Reprinted with permission from *Australian Family Physician*.

multivolume storage and retrieval of data not in immediate use. This strategy greatly expands the data-handling capability. Such a machine is a single-job type capable of handling all of the billing and accounting requirements of a group practice and, in addition, storing and sorting the data records on patients. This machine, however, requires the continuing personal handling of paper records by doctors and the services of a full-time computer operator to run the machine system, in order to handle data entry and retrieval in an efficient way as data are produced by the doctor and the ancillary staff.

More recently, development work has been done on an IBM system 34 with three screen terminals, at the consulting desk and the reception area, and a mobile matrix printer. This system has a central processor core of 64K, 27 megabytes of disk storage, and the capability of handling several extra screen terminals. This system is a multijob type, and provides the facility for a real-time on-line data-handling activity that allows control of the computer system from the consulting desk by several doctors at the same time.

HARDWARE REQUIREMENTS

A number of small computer systems now on the market are capable of handling the kind of applications required in private medical practice. However, there are also a large number of small systems available that, by virtue of one job facility, a small central processor, delayed work processing functioning, reduced screen VDU capacity, or limited file format functions, cannot handle the integrated activities of a medical unit.

Past experience has indicated that there are certain minimum requirements below which the function is severely limited, and staff cost savings are not possible and do not justify the capital or cash flow outlay.

The degree of complexity of processing and the total bytes of data held on-line in order to allow direct consulting-room access to current patient records, as well as accumulating record storage, requires a minimum disk data space of some five to seven megabytes of storage per doctor (five to seven million surface characters), a central core processor (arithmetic/logic unit) of at least 64K to allow access by five doctors and reception desk concurrently, the ability of the central processor to support at least five video screens for the machine system, and, in addition, the capacity to handle two printers simultaneously. These printers may be line or matrix printers, but need a minimum output of 120 lines per minute (line printer) or 120–140 characters per second (matrix printer). In addition, the system configuration should allow for a job queue to be held in order to prevent access delays, and a print spooling facility is necessary to prevent work from piling up when printer access is not immediate. This makes it possible to give priority to printing output and reports without altering the job access from each terminal screen, and also allows use of different sizes and types of preprinted stationery without interfering with the smooth running of the practice itself.

The number of tasks handled by an installed computer system in a medical practice is limited only by the ingenuity of the users themselves — assuming that a machine configuration has been chosen that is relevant to the work requirements of the practice.

The following functions have already been introduced and tested: accounting and billing; debit and credit analysis; business and personal tax schedules; transaction sorting of work done to analyze efficiency of time spent per month; sorting of monthly activities into benefit item order and postcode districts to assess population trends; family master record files; patient master record files; patient history files detailing obstetric history, pediatric history, family history, medication, vaccinations, allergies, problem lists, data base questionnaires for rapid medical record structuring; patient history profiles, either in part or in total based on the above files (these are accessed via the consulting room terminal or printed out for transfer); drug and toxicology registers cross-referenced to prescribed items; resource register of other medical personnel and ancillary paramedical services; ICHPPC code file for problem analysis; and preventive-care sorting for regular follow-up of smears and vaccinations.

Two other possible functions may be added to the above, namely, appointment scheduling and patient management problems for teaching purposes.

SOFTWARE

The kind of programs written to handle medical data processing in a private practice need to be considered from two aspects: billing and accounting, and medical record storage and retrieval.

As many readers are no doubt aware, the advent of small business computers has led to a demand for software programs that are customized to handle work in groups of industries where tasks remain the same, whatever the nature of the business. Thus one may obtain from the suppliers of hardware, system support packages that will handle all types of data processing in a general way. In addition there are software packages that supply machine access in a high-level computer language that will even make it possible for the first-time user without particular programming skills or experience to structure files for data storage, access and to process these files and produce controlled output of data.

Thus far the problem is not difficult. Added to this is the ready availability of program packages that will handle payroll, invoicing, parts and warehouse function, ordering, billing, etc.

However, to date most of the software packages available to the medical profession are geared to business or professional use and do not provide the special requirements of medical patient billing or organize and prepare the kinds of patient accounts that relate to medical benefit refunds from either government or insurance agencies.

A new software package needs to be written. This would then need to be used effectively on a cost-justified basis in order to warrant the introduction of computer systems into practice. This means planning a configuration that would, in fact, also be capable of handling medical data storage on a patient-by-patient basis to generate medical records.

Given such a possibility, simple efficiency would require that the accounting data be integrated with the patient medical records on a family basis; otherwise there would be a need to run two separate systems. This would require additional ancillary staff to handle the systems, immediately destroying the cost justification for the introduction of a computer that made the whole idea feasible.

So the problem begins to escalate. The design and writing of a group of computer programs that will handle the completely integrated requirements of a medical-practice data-handling environment is not (in spite of the claims of many software vendors currently showing interest in the potential medical market) something that can be run up in a few weeks for the practice on a particular hardware system. Such a system is now fully operational in the author's practice, and has required two and a half years of design, writing, and testing in a working practice environment.

Detailed Design

The purpose of the operating system as it now stands is to provide as integrated a set of functions as possible with as many of these as can be organized in the system, to be handled directly from the consulting room. This eliminates double handling of data and reduces the staff costs involved.

In addition, as much of the data processing as possible has been created as a machine task rather than a doctor or staff task, thus making maximum use of machine capability.

Medical Records

The main design criterion in this area was that of providing only sufficient structure to allow the computer to operate efficiently, and maximum allowance has been made for the individual doctor to use free-form English in the entry of data. Thus the following hierarchical medical record storage system is used: family master file; patient master file; data base; accounting detail; history files: problem list, obstetric, pediatric, family history, X-ray, laboratory, vaccination, allergy, medication.

Access to all of these files is by both direct entry and output, and by data transfer and chaining of files by the computer itself during entry of progress notes. The key to all of these files lies in the family number and terminal digit.

Thus each family in the practice is given a unique number which contains a practice number or doctor number to identify work done or work areas for later analysis of medical and accounting activities, and a family number group. To this is added a patient number to give identity to each individual; for example, doctor or surgery 01; family 1985; patient A father, B mother, 1 eldest child, 2 second child, 3 third child, and so on to 9 (10 being the exception).

In order to provide maximally rapid access to what becomes an enormous data base in a group practice, to eliminate the need to store any piece of data more than once, and to preserve confidentiality, the data files have a dependent hierarchy. The family file contains the family number. The patient file contains only the terminal digit as a key; all dependent history files are then accessed only by disk address and contain no direct data identifying them by person. This makes it possible for an outside epidemiologist to use files for research purposes without breaching confidentiality in any way. Data returning to the practice from various areas are entered into the dependent files by the practice receptionist from her own reception desk screen terminal.

Progress Notes

With the need, in the interest of efficiency, to control as much of the data system as possible from the consulting desk, the progress note entry containing day-to-day information becomes the most significant data structure. It acts as a central storehouse of material which may then be transferred and sorted by machine function by the use of simple codes contained within the note entry.

In order to allow for the individual note pattern of a particular doctor, allowance for a free-form entry must be made where possible. However, the nature of a computer system and the need for constant data control for both sorting and data transfer to other systems at some stage make it necessary to introduce at least a degree of rigidity into the progress note layout.

To ease the problem of rigidity, such terms as "objective" and "subjective" assessment have been used. However, this is rather too-free form and may create confusion in international usage while medical schools are still teaching a traditional note structure. Consequently a structure has been created that allows for both freedom and some rigidity.

The progress note is divided into the following sections, which are prompted for individually on the screen terminal: history (as told by the patient in summary); examination (as found by the doctor); WT, BP, urine; plans (either tests, opinion, or when to return); treatment (medications, with generic name, strength, doses/day); problem name (ICHPPC code); code (transfer code for problem lists); item no. (medical benefits schedule).

History. This is entered as a free-form summary of the story presented. After much experimentation, it has been found that 120 characters of data space provide the most flexible entry. This space may be exceeded in some psychological problems when a second progress note can be continued.

Examination. Free-form entry of findings and 120 characters of data space provide for most entries.

WT, BP, Urine. These are common and significant tests done most frequently during a consultation and may need to be sorted for later epidemiological studies. Entering them separately takes no longer and allows complete machine sorting.

Plans. This allows for aide memoire and also encourages one's thinking at the time of entry in a logical order.

Treatment. All medications are listed in the form – generic name, drug strength, doses per day – and a code is added for all long-term medication (e.g., hypertension), for transfer to the patient medical file. Using a constant order also permits easy access by the computer.

Problem Name. Problem coding saves space, and the machine will access the ICHPPC file for the correct titles for the codes at output time. Use of an international code also allows correctability of findings when one is publishing research material.

Code. A simple code is used to allow the machine to transfer data in a meaningful way to the problem file: (1) A new problem of major significance is transferred to the patient history file. (2) Continuing problem, so no new data are transferred. (3) Minor problem for transfer to a standby file for later research access. (4) Resolved problem so problem file is tagged, and the same problem name is used as a new problem if it arises again.

Item No. In order to allow direct transfer of accounts ledger and accounts master file entries, the medical benefits schedule number is used. The computer selects from other files the description and fee as well as the family and patient number and automatically updates all account files. This, as one can appreciate, saves enormously on labor cost. The data transferred may then be used by the machine to prepare an instant bill at the reception desk, or are stored until the month's end and then used to prepare monthly invoices automatically. Further analysis of the work function and its effective value may also be done at the same time in an automatic procedure, thus giving effective work and time analysis without any further time being used by doctor or staff. These analyses may then be outputted as required.

Cost saving in this area alone in a group practice may be enough to cover the total cost of the computer system.

The use of such a structure in a constant way rapidly generates a logical approach to each problem as it arises and greatly enhances one's patient management.

OUTPUT

So far in this chapter consideration has been given only to input, but the whole exercise becomes meaningless without rational output. This topic will be covered in two sections: medical records and accounts data.

Medical Records

This involves a complete suite of programs. The system has been designed to provide instant access to all data held on the disk by the doctor in the consulting room via his own screen terminal. At the same time, when required, the data may be printed out in hard copy for transfer to other doctors or hospitals with the patient.

This is done by a patient profile structure so that all or any combination of sections of the patient's medical record may be displayed in the following order: data base (drawn from family master and patient master file); problem list (in chronological order); medication (long-term only); obstetric (details of each pregnancy in chronological order); pediatric (birth, 6/52, 12/12, preschool examinations); family history; allergy; vaccination (in chronological order); x-ray (summary of reports); laboratory (and other tests); and progress notes (full detail in chronological order).

The above headings are held on the screen as a constant display, and the entry of the patient number provides the key to the data requested, which are then immediately displayed. As the last entry is displayed from the record files, the screen then prompts for a "Yes" or "No" entry for a progress note to be entered. If "No" is specified, the screen returns to the above layout for the next patient. If "Yes" is replied, the progress note information displays for data to be entered, and on completion again returns to the original layout for the next patient. The same profile may be obtained in printout for transfer to other medical areas.

Accounts

This is the area in which cost justification is most likely to become apparent, and, as a simple straightforward task with which the doctors and staff are familiar, is a good entry point to computer function. With careful initial planning of the machine configuration, later growth can be allowed for, and a medical records data system may then be introduced as a second stage of development.

In the case of instant billing, an allowance in design may need to be made for a two-printer system in order to permit constant use of a matrix printer at the reception desk. Thus, in an integrated system, the entry of a progress note at the consulting desk with its contained schedule benefit item number will immediately generate a detailed account at the reception desk and apply a debit to the general ledgers. If the account is then paid, a credit is applied and the ledger balanced automatically. Otherwise, the transaction is held in a file until month's end, and then an invoice is produced for mailing. Using such a running transaction file chained to a family master file allows highlighting of debtors in a simple fashion.

In addition, the month's transaction file may be used to analyze the work done per practice or per doctor and permits efficient adjustment of time and work functions throughout the practice activity. Access to the master files at the reception desk also provides ease of handling account queries either directly or by telephone.

In a group practice of five doctors, careful computer design should lead to a saving of up to two full-time staff wages or, alternatively, may allow two staff to be released for other duties. Growth in the practice size should not lead to any further costs in staff time.

PROBLEM AREAS

The first and most immediate of these problems is the cost of the hardware. An average group practice of five doctors will need a machine system of around $60,000 capital cost in order to handle a totally integrated system. Such an immediate capital outlay is unjustified. However, on a lease basis such a system will cost in the vicinity of $1480 per month over four years. In addition, engineering maintenance and system support software will cost some $400 per month. Added to this is the cost of leasing the software suitable for handling an integrated practice activity. This will cost an estimated $300 per month.

Thus the total monthly outlay is $2180. However, the saving in staff costs may be up to $1300 per month, and an enhanced efficiency in handling debtors should make it possible to cover a portion or all of the additional cost.

The increase in patient management through control of patient medical records and the access to significant research material not currently readily available more than justify any further cost. In addition, income-tax benefits will accrue from the investment allowance on capital equipment according to the internal revenue laws of the country, state, or province.

It is possible with modern small business computers to provide security code access to all levels of data within the system, and thus confidentiality is ensured. However, as most of these machines are designed to be also used as part of a computer network, confidentiality may more easily be breached. This problem of confidentiality in a computer network has not yet been solved, and until it is, individual in-house systems seem to be the only acceptable alternative.

With all computer systems the risk of data loss is always present, though fortunately rare. However, erasure or deletions of sections of data or even whole files may be done easily from the controlling terminal on the system. Provision must therefore be made for backup of all data onto an off-line storage system as new material is generated in order to allow restoration of data that may have inadvertently been erased. This may be done onto shelf stored diskettes or removable disk packs. The larger tape systems are probably too expensive for normal medical-practice use.

Provision must also be made in system design for the archiving of data not currently required on-line in order to release disk storage space for current data. This may best be done by hard-copy paper files printed off the machine which may be referenced and photocopied if data transfer is needed. Progress notes are a good case in point. They need to be held as a detailed entry on-line for some two years, but may then be stored off-line as an archived reference. The same applies to families or individuals who leave a practice or are deceased. Access to such off-line storage is quick and simple.

A common problem encountered in systems handling the large amount of data needed to be held on-line in a medical system is the delayed response time in accessing the data via each terminal. This is more a problem in software design, but may also be the result of not allowing a central processor core size large enough to service the arithmetic logic needs of the system when maximally active.

Designed properly, with the use of a large program suite run as a never-ending program on a multiple requesting terminal basis, there should not be a response time greater than two seconds in order to fill a large screen completely with data. Anything slower than this is unacceptable and needs for the software to be rewritten.

CONCLUSION

An attempt has been made to present the concept of a totally integrated medical computer system without elaborating on the technical details.

With the developing technology of a modern society, medical practice has a pressing need to handle its increasingly larger and more complex data more effectively than it does at present. The ingenuity of the profession should surely be equal to the task.[2]

REFERENCES

1. Day and Larsen: "Medical Record Computer System." *Med. J. Aust.,* Aug 1978.
2. Brandejs, J. F., and C. G. Pace: Physician's Primer on Computers, Lexington Books, Lexington, Massachusetts, 1979.

8

EXPERIENCE WITH THE ALPHA MICRO (AM100) IN A DOCTOR'S OFFICE: BILLING

Peter E. Levers, M.B., B.S., L.M.C.C., F.R.C.S.C. (Urol)

To the orderly mind used to the world of computational logic the average medical office is unrestrained bedlam. But does the doctor know he has a problem? Doubtful. The average solution is to get a new receptionist, hire a part-time hand or put more chairs in the waiting room.

Norman Ronis, M.D.[1]

HOW OUR SYSTEM WORKS

Computers have been shown to be cost-effective in business for years. A couple of years ago I set out to see if they could save time and money and increase efficiency in a doctor's office. Together with an experienced programmer, we have shown that the new generation of computers are cost-effective in doctors' offices, whether they are solo specialists as I am or solo family practitioners. The system that I use costs about $300/month or about $10 a day to purchase.

It has been predicted that by 1982[2] 25% of physicians will be assisted in their offices by a computer. I purposely selected the word assisted, for there will be others with computer-*run* offices until they heave the machines out of the window! A system that disrupts your office or puts you or your secretary in a straitjacket is worse than useless.

The AM 100 is small enough to be built into the shelving in an office or mounted in a small mobile trolley as I have it, yet it is powerful enough to do all the billing functions for one or several doctors and can be expanded to cope with a clinic. I would recommend that when more than two doctors are using the system simultaneously, they purchase a ten-megabyte hard disk.

The new larger AM 100 can be used to set up a service bureau type operation within a medical building containing the offices of individual doctors, each user having his or her own terminal and printer and sharing access to a central computer equipped with large 92-megabyte hard disks. This configuration has economic advantages but necessitates several doctors agreeing to join the system at the outset.

The computer is a fast, accurate, and stupid machinery. It stores, sorts, scrunches, and retrieves information quickly; complex and repetitive calculations can be carried out in a fraction of a second. However, it is not stupid if it is programmed properly and told exactly what to do and when; this takes sophisticated software, often requiring weeks of planning and months of programming. Although the cost of computers and memory is decreasing, the costs of programming are escalating.

Communication with the computer is through the video, TV-like screen and keyboard. This people/computer interface is the key to acceptance of the system in any office; and it must be people-oriented.

To develop computer systems for doctors' offices, one must not only believe in "blue sky" specifications but also be a born optimist, work like hell, and have the time and the patience of Job. Before running to your new computer and starting to program, which is a tremendous temptation, you must first decide exactly what it is meant to do and how it will fit into your office. There lies the first pitfall, for neither the programmer nor the physician is competent to overcome this hurdle alone — the physician because of a lack of programming expertise and time and the programmer because of a lack of intimate knowledge of either the medical practice as it is or the peculiar philosophy of physicians. Thus, close and continual cooperation of physicians and programmers is essential.

"Blue sky" specifications means going for broke. The program has to be flexible enough to cope with all the vagaries and intricacies of medical practice, so that the computer does not get in the way of either the physician or his or her secretary.

Our programmer spent several weeks in my and other physicians' offices and drew up a set of specifications that was passed by a cross-section of physicians in our area. Soon it became apparent that each physician wanted to do it his own way. This confidence in a physician's own decision, which is central to his ability to practice, is probably the rock on which many previous medical systems have foundered. The programmer circumnavigated this problem by building in multiple options that the physician himself can select on a system control screen.

Secretarial acceptance depends on ease of learning (three half days); minimal change in her job; and ease of use. To this end we use a "form fill" technique rather than the question and answer used on most systems.

The first screen that the secretary sees asks for the date and password. She can move the curser around any of the white areas, adding or changing information until she is happy with it. The computer then checks it and adds information it already knows, and then re-displays it for her approval.

To further save secretarial time, all data are entered only once. The date keyed once on the password screen is used on every bill, insurance forms, daily log, etc., without having to be reentered.

The main menu displays patients accessed by name (given name first). However, those practices using numerical files can access the patients by numbers.

To select a function (e.g., billing), the secretary just moves the curser and puts an X against it. This takes her to the billing screen. The program further saves her time by automatically providing the usual data, but allows her to override them if necessary.

Thus, to bill a patient in most cases she has only to type in name, diagnosis, and fee code. The computer fills in the rest of the information, allowing her to check it, and to change it if required. When she is satisfied with it, she presses the return key and hands the patient a complete statement in four seconds.

Entering a new patient is just as easy. If the patient's family is already in the computer, she simply keys in the family head's name. Otherwise she has to key in address, phone number, % of doctor's fee, and insurance number.

At the end of the day she prints insurance forms, in our case punched cards accepted by the Ontario Health Insurance Plan (OHIP), day log, backs up, and goes home. Our experience is that it saves 70% of her time.

Secretarial acceptance has been good. My own secretary thinks it is the greatest thing since sliced bread. She particularly likes the system's ability to sort out the Mac's and Mc's using the search screen which lists patients either alphabetically or alphabetically by families. Then by X-ing the appropriate patient she can immediately call up his or her record, billing, or accounts receivable screens. She can define her own fee schedule. She may use her own mnemonic coding for the item, then link it to the used fee code, and insert the standard fee. The computer will supply the physician's and insurance fee automatically. The fees are re-displayed for her approval or correction before being stored in the fee file.

Sending out monthly statements to patients is usually tedious and time-consuming with most manual systems. They rarely go out on time. However, with the computer it is a breeze. In keeping with the flexibility of the system the secretary can select accounts by age, amount outstanding, and/or type. Dunning messages can be keyed by the secretary, and the computer automatically selects the appropriate message, depending on whether the patient has received payment by his or her insurance company.

My secretary gets reprinted statements selected at her request automatically while she has her morning coffee.

Your secretary will tell you what she thinks of doing health care insurance reconciliations. The computer displays either an alphabetical or a numerical list of claims submitted prior to the cut-off date, and she types a comment against any that do not match the insurance list. The computer posts all the correct ones to the appropriate account, prints a list of the transactions on the daily log, and then allows her to review the incorrect accounts receivable records, post corrections, or resubmit accounts to the insurance carrier. The time and annoyance saved by this program alone make the cost worth it.

Selection of Alpha Micro. After the specifications were drawn up, we went looking for a computer that would keep us within the C$10,000–C$15,000 price range (about $300 a month for a solo physician) and also supply the power and speed required for sophisticated programs and be capable of expansion to allow multiple terminals, printers, and hard disks for groups of physicians. The computer had to be a reliable business machine, not an overgrown toy.

The choice of the alpha micro has turned out to be a happy one. The extended alpha BASIC has many useful file-handling attributes including indexed sequential files, with no restriction on the size or number of files. A COBOL-like data division permits sophisticated record description, and statement labels enable us to compile programs without line numbers. A disk-based compiler enables us to precompile our programs, some of which are over 1000 statements in 64K memory, and run them in 48K storage.

Writing programs is facilitated by the two-dimensional vue editor, and debugging is eased by the ability to run in interactive mode. There are many other nice software operating system features.

Cybernex (A) cooperated with us in designing a microprocessor terminal that can run in either local or remote mode, and has inverse video, protected fields at full intensity and a flashing curser.

Alpha (B) have continued to expand and improve their software and their hardware. With the advent of their block transfer board, we will run multiple terminal systems with this board and up to a 92-megabyte disk storage.

Reliability of the system is of prime consideration in every medical office.

We had some static electricity problems — which have been overcome using a three-dollar can of fabric static spray. The new Cybernex terminals now have plastic-coated keyboards. Variation in electric power voltages have been dealt with by reporting the problem to hydro or using a "Sola" voltage regulator. Disk errors are now a thing of the past. We have learned that floppy disks must be handled with care, and the disk used daily should be retired about every six weeks. A lot of our earlier problems were caused by mishandling the disks themselves — throwing them down on a dusty desk, bending them, even on one occasion leaving back-up disks in a car and literally cooking them.

At last we seem to have got all the bugs out of the system software; some of them were pretty obscure.

The last thing any physician can afford is to lose data. To this end a paper trace is kept. Bills and cards are on two-part forms and are checked against the daily log. The trial balance program checks the data on disk of every account and prints any unusual findings. A special data-check program examines every account. Data are maintained in a bidirectional daisy chain so that fouled data links can be recovered. Three programs enable us to directly examine the electronic data on the disk and correct any errors that may occur. Modems (telephone links) enable us to perform diagnostic tests on equipment and correct data problems remotely, thus saving down time.

FUTURE APPLICATIONS

The computer has also provided unexpected bonuses such as the word-processing capability used to write and edit articles, reports, and such. Currently, general ledger packages are available for the alpha (a new one that will match our billing programs), and appointment programs are in the works.

The most exciting and most difficult area is the storing of patient histories. Currently, this can be accomplished using the vue editor and storing the electronic equivalent of a paper chart on disk. This, unfortunately, uses up a lot of disk space, necessitating a lot of floppy-disk swapping or purchase of a 10- or 90-megabyte hard disk. On the other hand, the storing of restricted data, (e.g., demographic record) only puts the physician in a straitjacket. The efficient storage of medical histories and data is in the preliminary planning stage. I would be more than happy to hear from physicians who have given any consideration to this problem.

CONCLUSION

The alpha micro 100, which was developed as a commercial machine, has been shown by us to have sufficient power and reliability to be used in physicians' offices.

The software, which was designed and developed in conjunction with doctors in practice and has been, and is now, running in physicians' offices, can be used to advantage by any physician.

In my office prior to the computer a part-time secretary spent four full days (32 hours/week) doing the billing, rebilling, and insurance cards. She also spent five hours a week on the books. She can now process a week's work in four hours!

A study[3] for a University of Toronto thesis has demonstrated a cost saving of $19,000 over a five-year period for a group of three "opted-in" family physicians. (Note: OHIP is a government-run medical insurance plan in the province of Ontario. Physicians who bill their patients directly and submit a card to OHIP which in turn pays the patient, are known as "opted-out." Those physicians who bill the plan and are paid by the plan, are known as "opted-in." OHIP requires different-colored cards, depending on the mode of billing. At the present time a physician may bill some patients opted in, others opted out. Our system copes with these patients easily, as well as with patients with no insurance or Workmen's Compensation Board cases.)

REFERENCES

1. Ronis, Norman: "My Girl Sends Out My Bills." *Physicians Micro Computer Rep.* 2(3):38, 1979.
2. Brandejs, J. *Physicians Primer on Computers*, CMA, Ottawa.
3. Feldman, M. K., and M. W. Kologinski: "A Feasibility Study of Computer Assisted Family Practice Units." University of Toronto thesis, 1979.
4. Levi, R.: Personal communication.
5. Gel., R.: Personal communication.

9
IMPROVING CLINICAL PERFORMANCE IN GENERAL PRACTICE WITH A $1500 MICRO—SYSTEM

Robert A. Johnson, M.D., Ph.D.
Grasscroft, Oldham
United Kingdom

The problem with new technologies is that they tend to be both complicated and expensive. Enthusiasts new to the field tend to make exaggerated claims, to overlook deficiencies in the operating of the new techniques, and, however well intentioned, to bring the innovation into disrepute. Imagine how you would introduce the technology of the automobile. You are unlikely to start by persuading people to purchase say a Rolls Royce, or a Thunderbird; you would make much better progress if you were to start them with, for example, a Volkswagen "Beetle." A similar analogy holds with medical computing. The system described here is not as speedy or as sophisticated as many connoisseurs of computing might wish. On the other hand, for the beginner it is simple, basic, and cheap; and it has immediate practical impact on the general practitioner's work, without putting him or her to enormous, undue inconvenience, or disturbing too much his or her general pattern of work.

Until computers can be shown to make a positive, useful, and cost-effective contribution to everyday medical practice, their use will be restricted to administration and accounting. Questions of convenience, cost, and confidentiality must all be satisfactorily resolved, before tangible progress can be made toward using the computer as a vital clinical aid. What is becoming clear, however, is the urgency with which these problems must be solved: the sheer quantity of data threatens, by its very mass, to impair the quality of clinical care delivered by the general practitioner.

So far, the computer has been too costly or too cumbersome for everyday usage. This fact has tended to obscure the growing crisis in handling or processing information that already besets the general practitioner. Last year for instance as a general practitioner in the National Health Service, I received over two million words of information about drugs. In a 12-month period, I saw 4,196 patients on 11,365 occasions, and recorded 31,110 symptoms, for which I advised 18,243 treatments (see *Journal of the Royal College of General Practitioners*, 1972, Vol. 22, pp. 655–60). From computer analyses such as these I estimate that in the United Kingdom there will be approaching half a billion (0.5×10^9) symptoms every year, with perhaps five times as many in the United States. The number of prescriptions is equally astronomical, with their cost shortly becoming insupportable.

The microcomputer offers a chance to mitigate these hazards, while at the same time providing a unique improvement in clinical care that has not previously been available. But before it does so, it must overcome the very real, and in many cases entirely realistic, prejudices of the medical personnel who will be required to operate it. Unless the computer system itself is trouble-free, cost-effective, and easy for the unskilled to use, the potential benefits from computerization will remain stillborn. So many claims made in the past remained unfulfilled, and so many promises went unkept, that this discussion will be confined to a system that is operating at the present moment, in a general practice, without hidden subsidy, research grant, or other extra financial support.

The stark fact of the matter is, that unless the computer system can demonstrate not only its utility but also its ease of operation, no amount of computer expertise or skilled salesmanship will persuade the busy general practitioner to employ the system. Using myself as a guinea pig in this situation as it were, being a practicing general practitioner, I can clearly see the disadvantages inherent in using complex new technologies, and I am also too familiar with the constraints of time on general practice. In designing the system described, I have had these fully in mind. To begin, therefore, we may usefully consider what a general practitioner should expect from his or her record system, whether the records are in pen on paper, or on magnetic storage media via a computer. There is a full range of medical data processing: starting with the operation of appointment systems up to the full clinical record, including the possibility of reporting or recording unpredictable adverse drug side-effects. Undoubtedly the computer could have impact on all these activities, but in the first instance the need is for immediate application and simplicity of operation. The main contribution of the present system is described as a "General Risk Index," whereby patients known to be "at risk" are given future appointments at their time of attendance. Whether they keep their appointments or not is checked electronically. In a word, defaulters are caught with electronic precision. There are other aspects of the system that emerge as the general practitioner becomes more familiar with it.

One of the principal problems of medical records in general practice is that of "data decay." This term implies that only 10 or 20 percent of the data recorded at each patient contact can possibly have long-term value. Much of the information recorded is of a trivial and perhaps transient nature and will be of little or no value on future occasions. The difficulty is in knowing at the time how to sort the clinical wheat from the trivial chaff. When dealing with smaller microcomputer systems, the threshold point is lowered so that symptoms such as the common cold or trivial injuries are not included, since they do not represent a long-term potential hazard for that patient, and therefore do not warrant inclusion in a defaulter's file. Incidentally, the only alternative to this severe culling of clinical data at the input stage is to record the doctor/patient interchange in its entirety and analyze in retrospect. Only such totality of recording can ensure that the information, which may be required at a later date, has in fact been recorded at the time. This feature of medical practice forms the basis for my major medical computing research whereby every item of clinical relevance that transpired between myself and a patient has been recorded for the last decade. The above statistics on general practitioner work load were, for example, taken from analysis of a small portion of this research. Suitable microcomputers for operating this larger system may become available within the next year or two (indeed one has recently been offered for sale in the United States for $3500), but since it involves considerably greater inroads into the general practitioner's work routine, it will not be further considered here.

The problem of convenience or inconvenience is paramount. No physician is prepared to subject either self or staff to a series of untried procedures that consume an inordinate amount of time. Nor should one, since one's primary responsibility lies with the care of the patients, and unless any new activity that the physician undertakes can be shown to be for their benefit, it would be unwise and perhaps unprofessional to so indulge.

This is undoubtedly a major barrier to the wider use of computers. Generally speaking they have been regarded as mysterious, complex machines, whose use is restricted to those with special programming skill and training. These skills are not easily acquired, nor are they readily available to the working physician. Even those doctors prepared to embark on the expense of a computer system, at some cost to themselves in terms of time and effort, have found great difficulty in explaining to the programmers and systems analysts precisely, or as precisely as they can, what their clinical demands will be.

In fairness it must be said that to benefit from the full potential of computerization, clinical practice will require change; in the ultimate analysis a true marriage of medical practice with computer techniques will involve adaptation on both sides. However, in the initial case, and certainly for the system to be described here, the demands on the first-time user are minimal, and the feedback is immediate. Moreover, the benefit increases the more time the general practitioner puts into the system. Indeed it has been designed with this characteristic in mind. As with all new techniques the so-called learning curve operates; that is, the longer the system or the operation is repeated or continued, the greater the facility of those using it. This applies as much to computer systems as to driving cars or handling other complex pieces of machinery.

Apart from the problem of inconvenience there has been a general distrust on the part of the medical profession of newfangled gadgets, especially those with the glamorous ethos of the computer. In part this arises from an unfounded suspicion that the computer will ultimately displace doctors from the provision of medical care to their patients. Though without foundation, this view has in fact been encouraged by various practitioners of the computing arts, fully without justification in my opinion. Let us be clear what the computer consists of. In essence it is a series of on/off switches. The system described below uses the switches to form a classification system analagous to those employing cards with holes punched around their edges. The latter manual system of card sorting involves the cutting through of the hole at the edge of the card so that if a knitting needle or wire were pushed through a pack of these cards, only those with a selected item specified would remain, as on a specialized grid or sieve system. In essence that is what the computer does, though it can sort through "holes in the cards" at a rate of approaching 1/2 million a second and can deal with up to four billion types of classification.

The main feature of today's technological scene is the speed with which these processes occur. The range and quantity of the material thus analyzed is growing enormously in size while decreasing enormously in cost. The microcomputer employed does indeed sort through selected data in a matter of microseconds, that is, up to a million items per second, though it is necessarily limited in other respects, as we shall see. In one important respect the number of categories must be limited in a machine of this price. To be specific, there are 57 diagnostic categories, which include 10 that may be allocated on a local basis by each general practitioner user. Owing to the widespread use of three-digit classifications among general practitioners using the RCGP code or the ICHPPC code, provision has been made for including the latter.

Thus the inconvenience of the present system has been minimized, even though this has entailed some diminution in the scope of potential benefits. In the initial phase, for example, the general practitioner is required merely to give each patient a five-digit number to be written on the record file and also at the same time in numerical order in a large ledger forming the "number index." Again at the price range contemplated, a manual system such as this, with respect to identification numbers, is considerably cheaper, faster, and less labor-consuming than other alternatives.

The supposition that computers will displace the clinician fails, since only the latter can choose into which category an individual patient or clinical presentation should fall. There is every reason to suppose that the clinical performance of the general practitioner using such a system will be improved, but this is not to say that general practitioners or other clinicians will themselves be displaced by such a system. Indeed there are powerful theoretical reasons, too complex to go into here, that indicate that computers are unlikely ever to displace the human patient/doctor relationship satisfactorily.

The priority is therefore to convince the general practitioner that his or her method of practice will not be grossly inconvenienced or distorted by introducing a computer system. The costs in terms of time expended by the physician or the staff must be kept to a minimum. Once the concept of computerizing data handling has been established, then the way will be open for more refined and sophisticated techniques; but until this happy point is reached, more elaborate computing machinery merely confuses the issue and further frustrates the initial introduction of the computer into the uninitiated general practitioner's routine.

The other aspect of cost, namely in financial terms, again is a critical factor. My estimate is that in the United Kingdom there is an upper limit of £1,000, above which the ordinary general practitioner loses interest. Whether the same financial limitation applies in North America, I am less able to judge. It has been my experience in the United Kingdom, that interest in computers ceases once the realization dawns that the outlay will be above £1,000. This cost restraint ties in well with the above policy of minimizing the inconvenience to the orthodox pattern of general practice. It clearly limits the sophistication of the equipment available. Many computer specialists would find this limitation not only irksome, but in some cases totally intolerable. Most computer consultants would, for example, deplore the absence of a "floppy disc" and the lack of provision for "hard copy." However, since the average general practitioner has received an adequate medical training but little familiarity with computer technology, let alone terminology, he or she has little conception of what these recondite sounding items might be and, in particular, no conception of where they might fit in with his or her particular computer system or indeed the general practice routine.

It has been judged essential that general practitioners familiarize themselves with the basis of computing techniques at the simplest level, before becoming involved in more elaborate items of computing equipment. I have no doubt that once the implications of computerization have been grasped general practitioners will be in a position to judge the suitability of both these items, and will undoubtedly see how they can complement and augment their growing microcomputer systems. The model of computer chosen has been selected with the provision of additional facilities in mind.

This leads us to the review of the currently available machines in the price range specified. Of the cheapest systems available that do not require the doctor to manipulate a soldering iron or become entangled in the intricacies of hexadecimal language or assembler code, there are two: the Commodore PET 2001-8 at £550 in the United Kingdom, between $700 and $1000 in North America, and the Tandy TRS-80. The former machine was chosen for the following reasons. At the level of 8K it was cheaper than the TRS-80, and clarity of the visual screen on which the information is displayed is astonishing — indeed exceeds that of machines of a much higher price range such as those I use at Manchester University. It has the added advantage of providing lowercase letters, which makes for a great deal of clarity on the screen. It has full cursor control, which allows for editing input; that is, errors and mistypings may readily be corrected on the screen by the user with great ease. The 4K RAM available on the cheapest machines is insufficient for any adequate programs, whereas the 8K is just manageable.

Confidentiality is of crucial importance. Again we must refer to the actual context in which medical practice takes place. The patient describes to the doctor symptoms and other details that are the raw material upon which the physician bases any further action. This flow of data, originating from the patient, is vital to the continuation of medical practice. Anything that impedes it is detrimental. Should the patient cease to have complete confidence that the information supplied will remain with the doctor, and not be relayed on from the medical context to his or her employer, spouse, the police, or elsewhere, this crucial source of information will cease. The patient will color his or her descriptions to take account of this fact, thus distorting the raw material of medical practice and causing serious deterioration in the efficient functioning of medicine. I am strongly of the opinion that only totally decentralized computing facilities can be tolerated. Certainly this is the case with the currently described microcomputer system, but the same principle applies more widely. Not only are telephone or land lines expensive, but they are "leaky" from a security point of view, and as such may not warrant medical use. The present system therefore is entirely decentralized, the information available is stored on magnetic tapes or eventually discs, and these items can be protected with more security than is currently available with paper-based records.

So we come to the actual system. The simplicity of operation may be emphasized by describing briefly its installation. Reference has already been made to the number index, which is kept manually. It is currently quicker to search for a given identity number in a ledger manually than to load and unload small-capacity floppy discs. In any event the latter are not obtainable under the cost restraints of this system. Thus the computer system identifies all patients by five-digit identity numbers to a maximum of 65,000 patients. No names or addresses are included in the magnetic records, in view of their cost in terms of volume of storage.

The first 8K program to be loaded by the user is a display program which is designed to familiarize him or her with the machine, to provide confidence in controlling the program by typing in various control numbers, and, in particular, to establish and encourage the habit of pressing "RETURN" after each data entry.

The second program is also loaded from the inbuilt tape deck, and this is used to enter the patient's five-digit identity number, the date on which the patient attends, and one of up to 57 risk categories.

Figure 1 illustrates the first of the two input displays. It will be noted that the last ten items are local items; they are designed for use by the individual users for allocation to categories that are of special interest to them (e.g., the study of a particular drug, adverse side reactions, or any of a host of different clinical entities). It will be noted that numeric values have been inserted for systolic and diastolic blood pressures. Similar numeric values are recordable for weight in terms of grams and kilograms, and height in terms of centimeters. Once entered these data can of course be retrieved; thus patients in excess of a particular weight, or whose systolic or diastolic blood pressure falls within a

1	B/P	2	WEIGHT	3	HEIGHT
4	DRUG	5	VACCN. DUE	6	ANTE NATAL
7	'PILL'	8	IUD – 'COIL'	9	CRVX SMEAR
10	SMOKING	11	SOCIAL	12	STRESS
13	ADMIN	14	MISCELLANY	15	Local-ONE
16	Local-TWO	17	Local-THREE	18	Local-FOUR
19	Local-FIVE	20	Local-SIX	21	Local-SEVEN
22	Local-EIGHT	23	Local-NINE	24	Local-TEN

Type Number?

Type Number? 1 = B/P

? 256 SYSTOLIC

? 112 DIASTOLIC

NEXT DUE in

? DAYS

? 6 WEEKS

Next due on FRIDAY 26 OCT 79

PRESS 'RETURN'

Figure 1. Common and local conditions.

certain range, may be identified in a later program on that basis. Referring to the earlier analogy of the card with punched holes, these are the slots that may be used, and the sorting programs that follow are used to select various combinations or all combinations mentioned.

The 30 diagnostic categories on the second input screen have been selected for their value in pragmatic clinical care. Natural candidates are those disorders that need constant supervision such as endocrine imbalance, cardiac problems, respiratory ailments, and so forth; in each case patients under surveillance can be more effectively followed. The third program reads through the General Risk Index tape generated by this section of the system, and picks out those who have defaulted, and have not attended before the date due as recorded.

Clinical performance can thus be improved in the following ways. First, defaulters in a surveillance program can be captured. Intervals between attendance for individual patients can be monitored, and a rough gauge of the efficacy of treatment can therefore be made. A general analysis of the contents of a given practice can be tabulated by analysis of the General Risk Index tape and the clinician's method of practice modified accordingly. Prudent use of the "local" factors could involve study of, for example, different hypotensive drugs with an automatic follow-up and assessment, and impact on blood pressure levels on all the hypertensives entered on the G.R.I. tape. Similar work could proceed with different oral contraceptive preparations.

Several features of the system become clearer during its operation. They have been designed to minimize inclusion of errors, and to permit easy and reliable usage. For instance, the first working program opens with a title page on the screen which is replaced by the first entry page on pressing "RETURN." The instruction "type in today's date" appears on the screen followed by "? day, month and year." Despite the small size of memory available, these dates are checked in various ways, and should they be "invalid," then a message to this effect is printed on the screen, and the cursor returns to the space in front of "DAYS?" Dates such as 30 February or 31 April or September, or indeed 29 February in other than leap years are automatically excluded. As a further check, no date earlier than 1 January 1950 is permitted. If the date is "VALID," the screen shows this by printing "Today is Wednesday 30th May 1980." The principle here is that any numbers input must be translated, so far as possible, into letters on the screen. In this case the days of the week have been calculated from the numeric input.

Next to appear is the Index or Menu Screen. This allows the user to control the system by typing in numbers from 1 to 9 which lead to various parts of the system. The first essential is to identify the patient for whom the risk factor is to be recorded, and this is done by typing in 1. In fact, no other part of the program can be reached until the identity details have been entered. Input screen for identity details is similar to that for inputing the day. The identity number must consist of five digits — anything less is erased. For example, to enter 100 it is necessary to enter "00100." On pressing RETURN, provided the number is valid, the following appears to the right of the screen on the same line "ID — 00100." A further line has now appeared on the screen, namely, "Sex?" Here again anything other than a word beginning with F or a word beginning with M, is merely erased from the screen and the system will not progress further. In point of fact, since most data entered are numerical, and the Commodore computer has a single key-pad to the side, the numeral 1 has been used for male and 2 for female. Entry therefore of an appropriate character at this level, and pressing RETURN, produces on the screen to the right-hand side either "MALE" or "FEMALE" as appropriate, and then the word "BIRTHDATE?" followed by the word "DAY?" The same date check routine operates, though in this case days up to 1 January 1900 are permitted. Patients born earlier than 1900 are entered as though they were born on 1 January 1900. This is a compromise dictated by the size of the memory. Completion of the date of birth, provided it is a valid date, results in the words "born 11 MAR 55" appearing on the right of the screen opposite birthdate. The bottom line of the screen now reads "to correct type 1." This allows any of the items to be corrected. Typing one at this point and pressing RETURN brings the cursor up the beginning of the identity number at the top of the screen. If no further change is required, repeatedly pressing RETURN brings the cursor successively down through identity number, sex, day of birth, month of birth, year of birth, and back again to the bottom line. If 1 is not typed at this point, or RETURN is pressed without entry, the user is returned to the Menu page, which now displays at the top "Today is Thursday 27th September 1979, Patient's ID is 00100 Male 11 Mar 55," followed by the Menu or Index as before. Risk conditions can now be entered either Common or Local as per Figure 1, or Diagnostic Risks or indeed a three-digit code as mentioned before. It should perhaps be mentioned again that on input of the three-digit code the actual code used is not translated on the screen, again owing to shortage of memory and limitations of storage media. Nevertheless, the commonly used three-digit codes can be included at this juncture, and they are stored as the "X-CODE."

On each occasion the date next due can be entered as through Figure 2. After each date entry the user is returned to the Menu page. On typing 5 on this page and pressing RETURN the data input up to that point is displayed on the screen shown in Figure 2.

As seen in Figure 2, the patient's identity number appears on the top left-hand side of the screen followed by sex and date of birth and today's day and date. The subsequent lines are numbered at the extreme left in reverse field. In the center of the screen the meaning of the digits to be stored is translated for

00100 MALE 11 MAR 55 THURSDAY 27 SEP 79

1	1	B/P
2	2256	SYSTOLIC
3	3112	DIASTOLIC
4	29167	DUE 8 NOV 79
5	43	HEART
6	29153	DUE 25 OCT 79
7	1211	X-CODE
8	29293	DUE 13 MAR 80

TO DELETE ANY OF ABOVE TYPE 'D'?

Figure 2.

the user to edit if necessary. Blood pressure, systolic, and diastolic readings are shown, and the patient is seen to be due on 8 November 1979. A heart condition that the patient also has is due for review on 25 October 1979. The "X-code 1211," which is not further translated, is due to reattend on 13 March 1980. The bottom line on the screen asks whether any of the above lines require deleting, and if they do, the user is requested to type in "D." This is a double-check device that prevents data from being erased in error. If D is typed in and RETURN pressed, then the next line to appear is "To Delete type in number?" and any number then typed in will cause the line of that number to be erased. Thus should an error have occurred in any of the data entered, the user has this opportunity to correct and reinsert it via the Menu or Index page.

When satisfied with the data for that patient, the user may press RETURN to go back to Index page, where 6 may be typed to enter details of the next patient in a similar fashion. Typing 7 on this page allows the data thus entered and edited to be stored on tape under the heading "General Risk Index, 27th September 1979, page 1."

Typing 9 on the Index page allows the user to exit from that program, permitting him or her to load the third program, which catches "defaulters." Here the GRI is read in and analyzed to a range of dates specified by the user. Again the system has been designed to be as foolproof as possible; for instance, it is not possible to get through to the Index page without inserting the day on which the analysis is being conducted. Again on reaching the Index page the first requirement is to set the date range; this is accomplished by either typing 1 or simply pressing RETURN. This step has the effect of preventing other parts of the system from being used before the range has been set. The range is specified in either days, weeks, or months, going backward in time from today's date, and the screen on which this information is entered is headed by today's date. On entry of a given range and pressing RETURN, the screen then shows "Range to be screened is from Thursday 9th August 1979 to today." On pressing RETURN the Index page again appears, and it now contains the same information as the preceding screen, namely, "Range to be screened Thursday 9th August 1979 to today."

The stage is now set for entry and analysis of the "GRI tape." This is accomplished by typing in 2 and pressing RETURN. The procedure that appears on the screen is "Be sure tape is ready and demagnetized." The importance of demagnetization was brought home by difficulties with earlier models for this system, where the tape recording heads became magnetized with unpleasant ease. On pressing RETURN the instruction then appears on the screen "Press play on tape 1." This allows entry of the GRI tape previously recorded in the earlier program. The heading is "Recording Tape GRI 30th August 1979, 32 lines." The actual numbers entered are printed on the screen and remain there until RETURN is again pressed. On pressing RETURN the word "ANALYSING" appears on the screen, followed in a short time by something similar to Figure 3.

In Figure 3, the top line of the screen is day and date again, followed by the range to be screened, and then the patients, in order, who fall within this category. The first such patient has the code number 13261 — she is female and was born on 24 January 1953. She attended the surgery on 29 August and was due to return on 30 August for reassessment of asthma. The second patient similarly attended a day later and was due for attendance on 13 September, in this case for reexamination of his blood pressure. The third patient was born in 1933, as can be seen, and was due to attend on the 27th, namely on the same day on which this particular analysis was being conducted. In this case the patient had had a mild stroke, had made a good recovery, and was about to return to work. The last line on the page gives the opportunity to delete any of the individual patients who may either have already attended on their due date or may have been excluded for other reasons. Such patients' details as the user allows to remain can now be stored on a further tape, whose color tag is yellow and whose use is further storage of those patients screened on this particular date range.

The fourth program to be loaded is essentially similar to the one just described, but instead of screening for "defaulters," this program screens the GRI tape for individual clinical items selected at the time by the user, using a screen similar to those shown in Figure 1. It may be noted that actual blood pressure readings can also be sought out, using this particular program, thus grouping all patients in a given category. The nature of identification of these patients is directly similar to that already described, namely, their identity number, sex, and date of birth, and naturally the condition for which they are being screened and the date on which they initially attended, as recorded on the GRI tape. The size of

TODAY IS THURSDAY 27 SEP 79.

RANGE to be screened —

THURSDAY 9 AUG 79 — TODAY

| 1 | 13261 ID Number FEMALE born 24 JAN 53

29   AUG 79 = Date ATTENDED

30   AUG 79 = Date DUE for ASTHMA

| 2 | 3110 ID Number MALE born 2 OCT 16

30   AUG 79 = Date ATTENDED

13   SEP 79 = Date DUE for B/P

| 3 | 10556 ID Number MALE born 9 JAN 33

30   AUG 79 = Date ATTENDED

27   SEP 79 = Date DUE for C/BRAL + C

TO DELETE ANY OF ABOVE TYPE 'D'?

NOTE: Boxed items represent reverse field.

ASTHMA

Figure 3.

memory available limits the number of combinations of such categories that can be screened in this manner. However, local categories may be combined with others (e.g., use of a particular drug and its effect on the blood pressure reading), thus permitting detailed research projects.

The fifth program permits linking of references to the same patient to be collated. Again the 8K memory places some restriction on this, but the user can allocate the available memory as he or she best wishes. Ideally, all references to the same patient should be accumulated in one spot. The remaining five sections of the system relate directly to the "age/sex register." Program six, for example, allows the construction of this register on a similar basis to that for the General Risk Index, in that date of birth, sex, and ID number of each patient are entered and may be edited as before. Program seven allows the sorting of the age/sex register into a variety of age/sex groups chosen by the user at the time. Program eight is of particular relevance only to British general practitioners working in the N.H.S., since it relates to "capitation fees." If any health service requires computerization, it must be the N.H.S., since it has become a bureaucratic jungle. Among the several methods by which a general practitioner is paid is the "capitation fee," which has three values, depending on the year in which the patient was born. The somewhat byzantine methods by which the capitation fee is calculated have successfully been encapsulated in a small segment of this particular program. The age groups and indeed the capitation fees are shown graphically and numerically. Program nine allows entry of tapes with identity numbers resulting from any of the preceding programs to be sorted into numerical order for ease of reference back to the patient's name and address, via the manually compiled number index, which, as may be recalled, has been kept in strict numerical order regardless of the name or other identifying details of the patient. The normal method of filing gives similar manual reference from the patient's name in alphabetical order to his or her identity number. Program 10 allows the age/sex register to be updated by deleting those who have left the practice area and inserting new additions to it.

From the detailed description just given, some principal deficiencies become clear. The first is the size of memory. This is the most easily rectified problem, since electronic memory is relatively cheap, and the machine in question can be upgraded for a few hundred dollars to 32K. This would considerably ease the problem of programming and extend the versatility of the system. Additional equipment, notably a second cassette deck, would allow the sorting and storage of updated files to be run automatically. These two items are relatively inexpensive, though it should be pointed out that together they increase the price of the basic machine by almost 50%. Even greater proportional price increases are required for the next increments in equipment. The most useful would probably be a printer, but reliable printing devices suitable for use with a microcomputer cost more than the original equipment itself, often up to £1,000. Similarly, with a disc unit the price again exceeds that of the original outlay.

It may freely be conceded that a computer system lacking a printer or a disc unit is very much a "poor man's" machine. Nevertheless, the price of such systems, *excluding* programs or software, is at least three times the price quoted for this sytem including software. The real problem is not whether the thing can be done, but whether it can be done at a price in terms of cash and inconvenience that the doctor will bear. Although each may well extend the sophistication of the system, it also increases the complexity and inconvenience to which the user is subjected. In particular, the floppy discs currently available for microcomputers have shown a number of unreliable features and difficulties of implementation.

In dealing with beginners in this complex field, the advantages of a cassette storage medium, with which the user is likely to be familiar from the audio field, probably outweigh the advantages in computer facility offered by the disc. As noted above, once the user has become familiar with the value of computation, there is nothing to prevent him or her from expanding the system to include these more expensive items of equipment, which will undoubtedly extend the speed and sophistication of the computing system. But until the initial "culture shock" has been breached, it would seem prudent to keep the system simple, basic, and cheap, while nevertheless producing practical results that are unobtainable by conventional or manual means.

The improvement in clinical performance for a general practitioner using the system arises principally from superior data processing. It allows him or her to automate vaccination schedules and the contraceptive users register, including whether patients are on oral contraceptives or intrauterine devices; it allows the physician to see that all defaulters are caught, a facility not available using cumbersome manual methods based on paper and card; further, it permits analysis of those patients particularly at risk and even basic research into the patterns of morbidity in the practice, even to the extent of detecting those patients who attend more frequently than others. Drug usage can be monitored, and limited assays of efficacy can be undertaken in particular with respect to hypotensives and weight loss regimes. This analysis of clinical performance brings the general practitioner information that is otherwise unobtainable, and which may allow modifications in the work routine to maximize clinical efficiency. It allows an overview of the physician's practice, for more efficient prophylaxis or defensive medicine, and in general lets the physician know more about what he or she is doing than was known before.

Referring to my opening paragraph, this microcomputer system will initiate an otherwise sceptical general practitioner into the exciting possibilities of clinical improvement that computerization holds. The story is told of a man who, on hearing of the automobile, asked "What would I need one for? I never walk more than three miles a day." Such an attitude is entirely appropriate for many of today's general practitioners, since the machinery available for them has little direct relevance or immediate impact on their contemporary situation. It is notable that motor transport only became available on a wide basis with the model-T Ford, and it is precisely this role that the microcomputers of today fulfil. Undoubtedly, the system described is a basic and rather limited one. Nevertheless, it would give reliable use for perhaps the next ten years, and provide a fundamental education for the working clinician on the assets to be had from computerization. In particular, it will prepare him or her for the other logical extreme, namely the total displacement of paper from the clinical records, thus allowing the electronic analysis not only of the 50 or so items mentioned here, but of every symptom, sign, diagnosis, and treatment that forms the basis of major clinical research work — a concept that will undoubtedly gain wider appeal once the psychological barrier of the computer has become overcome, though certainly not before.

The writer wishes to thank Professor Metcalfe, of Manchester University, England, for his timely advice. Developments are under way to adapt the system for use on a TANDY TRS 80.

10
DOCTOR'S OFFICE COMPUTERS IN THE GERMAN HEALTH SYSTEM

Erhard Geiss
Zentralinstitut für die Kassenärztliche
Versorgung in der
Bundesrepublik Deutschland
Fed. Rep. of Germany

THE LEGAL AND POLITICAL BACKGROUND

The type of EDP systems used in a doctor's practice will be determined by the general political environment regarding health policy, and by the actual contractual and legal rules for ambulatory treatment in the particular country. The health care services in the Federal Republic of Germany lay the main responsibility for both curative medicine and the entire range of preventive medical care measures on the 57,000 authorized doctors in individual or group practices (Figure 1). The methods of work in this area — from the data-processing point of view — are subjected only to general and broad legal or statutory guideline regulations, which are then crystallized into concrete and detailed form by agreements, contracts, and informal agreements within the self-governing bodies.

The rules and methods of ambulatory treatment as currently practiced represent a system that has grown up within one generation and is oriented to conventional methods of communication and documentation. To obtain benefits from rationalization effects resulting from the introduction of new information technologies, it is necessary as a precondition to make far-reaching changes in both the procedural organization and the formal contractual regulations (Figure 2). As a consequence, the demonstrated functional effectiveness of computers for doctors is, in terms of the total organizational picture, not the end, but rather the beginning of a demonstration project for improving both performance and the information situation in this area.

The federal government is supporting the medical profession in independent, wide-ranging field tests to investigate in closer detail those procedures in a doctor's practice that are capable of being rationalized by the use of EDP with

Doctors in the F.R. of Germany (1978)

In free practices	57,509	38%
In hospitals	63,354	42%
In science/administrations	9,948	6%
Not practicing	20,754	14%
	———	———
Total doctors	151,565	100%

Health Insurance Coverage (1978)

Population of F. R. Germany	61.3 Mio	100.0%
– general medical scheme	55.3 Mio	90.2%
– private or other coverage	5.8 Mio	9.5%
– not insured	0.2 Mio	0.3%

Figure 1. Medical profession and health insurance.

respect to their effects, the profile of procedures, services performed and prescriptions, and the associated reduction of costs and increase of service performance, including the concrete advantages in the care of the patients. Apart from the analysis of the factors involved in improving the functionality of the health care provided, it is also intended to produce a list of measures necessary for adapting and matching the conventionally organized data and information environment to EDP-user systems. This also applies to the behavioral interactions between the patient, or the medical personnel, and the EDP system. The flows of data between the doctor's practice and the Kassenärztlicher Vereinigung (Association of General Medical Scheme Doctors) and the Krankenkassen (General Medical Scheme Insurers) must also be subjected to constructive critical analysis from the same standpoint.

If the use of EDP in ambulatory treatment succeeds in reducing the costs incurred by or induced by doctors by fractions of a percent, this project will be profitable to the economy as a whole.

STATE OF DEVELOPMENT OF A COMPUTER FOR DOCTOR'S PRACTICES

The reduction in size of EDP systems and the reduction of their unit capital cost make computers attractive to almost all the independent professions in Germany. Ambulatory medical care is also a field in which the penetration of EDP-supported

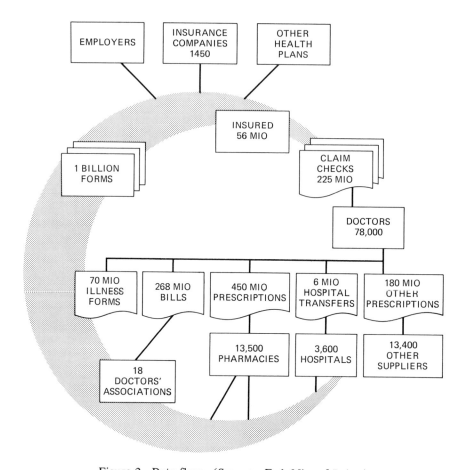

Figure 2. Data flow. (Source: Fed. Min. of Labor)

procedures is unstoppable. In the meantime a large proportion of the shared-practice laboratories and a number of group practices and associated practices are using EDP for partial technical or administrative purposes.

In the Federal Republic of Germany there are currently about 20 firms — manufacturers, software firms, or so-called systems firms — supplying or developing EDP systems for the medical market (Figure 3). These systems without exception employ design concepts based on a few individual forms of medical practice, are tailored to certain particular hardware elements, and are very restricted in their range of functions. Thus the core of the administrative work in the doctor's practice, viz., the quarterly invoice to the Kassenärztliche Vereinigung, receives no data-processing assistance from any of these systems.

Hardware of Implemented Doctor's Office Computers

Data General Eclipse
Hewlett Packard HP 250
IBM System/1
Digital Equipment LSI 11, PDP 11/34
PLESSEY MICRO I
NCR 820
SIEMENS
QUANTEL
UNIVAC UTS 700
NIXDORF

Figure 3. Hardware-spectrum.

On the other hand, an EDP system tailored to the needs of the doctor's practice can be put together from the large number of hardware and software elements offered. This freedom in choosing component parts has been found very favorable by the Zentralinstitut, and this factor, as well as its independence of short-term market successes, has considerably fostered the flexibility of the demonstration project.

THE RESULTS OF GOVERNMENT-SPONSORED PROJECTS

At the same time, the preparatory work necessary to provide the doctor's practice with a working technical system is no less difficult. These problems must be solved at a prior time, to provide an adequate basis for the reorganization. The Zentralinstitut has therefore over a period of four years developed and carried out practical tests on various computers for doctors, within the framework of a research project under the financial sponsorship of the Federal Ministry for Research and Technology. The first system was demonstrated publicly in 1975, for the ophthalmology specialist group. At this time it was recognized (and this was confirmed by a study trip to the United States) that decentralized EDP systems offered considerable technical, economical, and motivational advantages over a central data-processing organization. In its early utilization of process-control computers the Zentralinstitut was a logical step ahead of the trend that began in subsequent years toward mini- and micro-computers.

Meanwhile a consolidated system concept is available, the mature third generation of computers for doctors, that provides data-processing support for the central core functions common to the procedures of all doctors' practices. This development has also taken into account the results of experience in terms of space, air-conditioning, and temperature requirements and also the degree of cost loading that the doctor's practice can tolerate. The program and data-file systems are independent of one another in their content. The modular structure of the system makes it independent of both the structure of the practice and of the medical specialty in which it operates. The experience gained on pilot tests with doctors has shown where the practical points of friction (which could not be foreseen in advance) with existing conventional procedures occur, which can fully counteract the rationalization advantages produced by the use of computers.

Under this group of problems fall questions of the identification of the patient, his proof that he is insured, the design of forms, and their coding with "speaking code-keys." This interface problem is also relevant inside the practice, since a variety of daily procedures must still be carried out manually. In this connection the question arises as to what extent, both qualitatively and quantitatively, the computer can be admitted to consulting and treatment rooms.

OPERATIONAL EFFECTS ON AMBULATORY TREATMENT

An analysis carried out by the Zentralinstitut in which 50 doctors were questioned as to what they expected of the use of computers gave a largely homogenous picture of their opinion of the rationalization effects (Figure 4).

An important argument in favor of the use of modern information technology in doctors' practices is the increased "self-responsibility" of the patient, which means that he requires detailed information on the cause of the illness or complaint, on its progress, and on the best treatment. It may be necessary in the future to provide the patient with individual instructions as to what he should do, in printed form, in addition to the personal discussion with the doctor.

On the other hand, the doctor is under pressure to limit costs. The doctor's practice can only ensure conformance with the system if it has available, to a greater extent than hitherto, price-comparison information, cost-effectiveness analyses, and performance statistics. The feedback provided by the bookkeeping results from the Kassenärztliche Vereinigung, pharmacists' central invoicing departments, and the associations of health insurers is currently produced with a time lag of four to six months, which makes a timely reaction by the practicing physician, who generates these costs, impossible. A computer for the doctor's practice can provide an up-to-date and detailed profile of services and costs.

Scientists and health politicians have in recent times been calling more strongly for feedback of information — particularly with regard to preventive medicine (early detection of illnesses) and follow-up care (oncology) — between the various points at which ambulatory and in-patient treatment is provided, with the patient's active participation. This can hardly be provided on a broad basis in ambulatory care without the increased use of EDP. Controlled invitation models,

Expected Improvements by Computers for the Physician's Office

	Yes
Efficient documentation	76%
Substantial time savings	68%
Accurate/transparent billing	62%
Automated form & reports	62%
Operational advantages	58%
Advantage for patients	50%
Increasing capacity	48%
Reduction of cost	38%
Reduction of personnel	34%
Faster findings/diagnoses	18%

Expected Constraints by Computers for the Physician's Office

	Yes
Monthly computer expenses of $\leqslant$ S 1200 tolerable	84%
Negative reaction of personnel	24%
Negative reaction of patients	8%

Figure 4. Expected effects of computer application. ZI-analysis in 50 solo-practices, 1976.

checking up on follow-up care appointments, and also various forms of quality assurance by means of statistical comparisons can only be provided at acceptable cost by using data-processing support. However, for this it is necessary, in view of the largely high-volume nature of curative treatment in the doctor's practice, for a functionally competent basic system to have already found acceptance.

PROBLEMS OF INTERFACING WITH THE CONVENTIONAL ORGANIZATION

The use of computers in the doctor's practice takes the form of substituting for, or modifying, repetitive procedures that have been carried out manually and on paper. The EDP system should be regarded by the persons involved as a "multiplier" of human working capacity (searching, storing, finding, comparing, evaluating). For each person involved, this should mean that he can improve the quality of his work, or can increase the scope of his function in the health service (Figure 5).

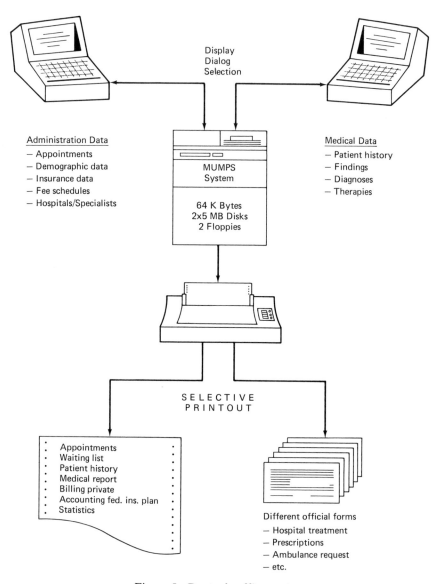

Display
Dialog
Selection

Administration Data
— Appointments
— Demographic data
— Insurance data
— Fee schedules
— Hospitals/Specialists

MUMPS
System

64 K Bytes
2x5 MB Disks
2 Floppies

Medical Data
— Patient history
— Findings
— Diagnoses
— Therapies

S E L E C T I V E
P R I N T O U T

- Appointments
- Waiting list
- Patient history
- Medical report
- Billing private
- Accounting fed. ins. plan
- Statistics

Different official forms
— Hospital treatment
— Prescriptions
— Ambulance request
— etc.

Figure 5. Doctor's office system.

Since different practices have differing methods and emphases, adequately flexible interfaces must be adopted between conventionally organized procedures and a unified technical system design concept. The high degree of flexibility and adaptability of ambulatory procedures at changing problem points must not be narrowed by the use of EDP, but should, on the contrary, be increased by the higher degree of "transparency" of both medical and administrative procedures.

The acceptability of EDP-supported system concepts, which to the extent of about 80% consist of a dialogue between the consulting-room assistant and the EDP system, depends in routine use on ease of operation and reliability. Among the doctor's-practice computer designs on the German market, the tendency toward a single system concept applicable to all different medical specialities, which (on grounds also of cost and of learning to use it) can be implemented in stages, is only slowly asserting itself.

The typical hardware for the doctor's office contains one display terminal each in the reception area and in the secretary's office, where the process data can be collected from the (still manual) medical procedure documentation. The organizational link between the EDP system and the conventional data system is an internal patient key-code. The doctor himself requires no direct contact (keyboard) with the EDP system.

ARCOS — A COMPUTER FOR DOCTOR'S PRACTICES BY THE ZENTRALINSTITUT

For the Zentralinstitut the market situation is such that, based on the total individual-practice organizations, there exist common procedures that can be isolated. The result of this analysis, in the form of an EDP system, is the Standard ARCOS system.

Apart from offering complete and fault-free data recovery by simple operator actions, the system also offers direct reasonableness checks on the data, with an on-line correction facility. In Standard ARCOS 30 different types of patient information (files) can be manipulated using only four commands. A series of items of information available by pushing buttons permit detailed or overall survey of the individual treatment case or of the performance of the practice. The storage of data is so organized that even for data extending over several quarter-years only a single operation is necessary. At the same time all data that are no longer current (e.g., performance data) are put in secondary storage.

The difference between patient-oriented tasks (the everyday work of the practice) and text-oriented tasks, (the relatively infrequent maintenance of text and key-code files) is important. The type of operation is determined directly after the system is called up.

Using the initial letters of the desired functions (4) and the desired types of information (30), the operator has a simple but powerful set of around 80 commands at his disposal (Figure 6). The syntax is always the same:

[function] ⊔ [type of info.] ⊔ [text   1] \ . . . . . [text x]

Independent of the type of hardware, the system can be extended on a modular basis to increase its power several-fold. An OCR-B reading pen may be connected for routine data input or recall. The printer can be used for either continuous stationery or individual forms.

ARCOS is written in MUMPS (Massachesetts General Hospital Utility Multi-Programming System, ANSI Standard X 11.1-1977), which is a data bank system

Function / Type of Info.	Input	Display	Printout	Correction
1 Patient ID				
2 Demographic data				
3 History				
4 Findings				
5 Diagnoses				
6 Therapies				
7 Risk factors				
8 Notes				
26 Statistics				
27 Billing				
28 Practice parameters				
29 Sort/Merge etc.				
30 Copy/Restart etc.				

Figure 6. ARCOS commands.

designed for multiple access and includes the operating system and a higher-level programming language. The advantages of MUMPS lie primarily in the simple handling of texts — both in the development stage and also if the system is later extended.

The separation of the operating and data-holding system, independent of the software provided, which is in each case specific to a particular office, has major advantages. By using the MUMPS software, the ARCOS system is largely independent of a particular manufacturer, and shows considerable promise for the future, particularly in the direction of using modern microprocessors (Figure 7).

The Zentralinstitut's field test is being observed with considerable interest by doctors in practice, EDP manufacturers, and systems firms. It is anticipated that this project, financed by the German Doctor's Association and supported by the federal government, will become the cornerstone of a new sector of the data-processing market.

All the regional Kassenärztlichen Vereinigungen (Associations of General Medical Scheme Doctors) have formed a coordinating committee for "EDP in the doctor's practice," to enable the two-way data flows between the doctor's practice, the Kassenärztliche Vereinigung, the Federal Kassenärztliche Vereinigung, the General Medical Scheme health insurers, etc., to be dynamically matched and adjusted to the utilization of new information technologies.

Artronix: PC-12/770, Modulex
Burroughs: 1726, B 6700
Data General: Eclipse, NOVA, MicroNOVA
Digital Equip. Corp.: LSI-11, PDP11, PDP10
Ferranti
Harris
Hitachi
IBM: System /1, System 360/370
Intel: 8080
Microdata: Express
Modcomp
Motorola: 6800
Oki Electric
Philips: P800
PRIME
Tandem

Figure 7. Hardware for MUMPS. (Source: *MUG Quarterly,* Feb. 1979)

INTERNATIONAL COMPARISON

Although the health care systems in different countries exhibit very basic differences, the international state of development shows a number of similar doctor's-computer developments. In the first instance the basic administrative functions in the doctor's practice have been developed for applications modules ready for the market. The ABC system (Appointment, Billing, and Cumulative Patient Profiles), which has been realized by the Canadian Medical Association on various different computers, corresponds to the basic core functions of the Zentralinstitut's Standard ARCOS. The U.S. Project CAPO (Computer Aids for the Physician's Office), which has been tested mainly on doctor's common facilities, corresponds to some medical documentation functions of ARCOS as well.

Solutions for the worldwide needs for drastic reductions of cost expansion in medical care, for improving the interdisciplinary communication, and to increase the efficiency of human work and intelligence do not seem feasible without intensive EDP support — especially at the point of primary service.

BIBLIOGRAPHY

Bolt, Beranek and Newman, Inc.: "A Final Summary Report on the CAPO Project. An Assessment of the Utility of Computer Aids in the Physician's Office." Report 3096. Cambridge, Massachusetts, 1974.

Brandejs, J. F.: "Computer Assisted Physicians Offices." *Health Commun. Informatics* 5(2): 69ff., 1979.

Brandejs, J. F., M. A. Kasowski, and M. W. L. Davis: "Information Systems, Part IV: What the Computer Can Do for the Primary Care Physician." *J. Can. Med. Assoc.* 113: October 1975.

Bundesanzeiger, B. No. 148, P. 2, August 1973.

De Dombal, F. T., and F. Grémy (eds.): "Decision Making and Medical Care: Can Information Science Help?" *Proceedings* of the IFIP Working Conference. Amsterdam: North-Holland, 1976.

Digital Equipment Corporation: *PDP 11 Software Handbook.* Chapter 8: "Digital's Standard MUMPS-11," pp. 193ff. Maynard, Massachusetts, 1978.

Geiss, Erhard: "Arztcomputer in den USA: Eine Studienreise." In *Online-adl-nachrichten,* No. 4, pp. 279ff. Köln, 1977.

Geiss, Erhard: "EDV in der Medizin." Gastkommentar in *Bürotechnik,* No. 11, p. 50. Baden-Baden, 1978.

Geiss, Erhard: "EDV in der Praxisverwaltung — eine Bestandsaufnahme: Der Arzt-Computer läßt auf sich warten." *In Arzt und Wirtschaft,* No. 22, pp. 22ff. Stuttgart, 1978.

Geiss, Erhard: Arzt-Computer Grundstufe. Basis-ARCOS-Einführung. Köln, November 1978.

Geiss, Erhard, F. W. Schwartz, Rolf Brüning, and Leo Heinen: DOMINIG Teil III. Informationsverbund für niedergelassene Ärzte and sonstige an der ambulanten Versorgung beteiligte Einrichtungen unter Benutzung eines zentralisierten DV-Systems. Köln, September 1976.

Henley, R. R., Gio Wiederhold, et al.: *An Analysis of Automated Ambulatory Medical Record Systems*, Vol. 1: *Findings*: Vol. 2: *Background Material*. Technical Report 13(1). National Center of Health Services Research, Health Resources Administration, Rockville, Maryland, USA, June 1975.

Hirche, Wolfgang: "Der Computer erobert die Praxis." In *Selecta*, No. 22, pp. 2096–2100, May 1978.

Kark, Gerhard: " 'Gesundung' des Gesundheitswesens durch Rationalisierung." In *Online-adl-nachrichten*, No. 9, pp. 674ff., Köln, 1978.

Lönneker, Walter: "Größeres Wirkungsspektrum durch Computereinsatz." In *Bürotechnik*, No. 11, pp. 24ff. Baden-Baden, 1978.

Lönneker, Walter: "Datenverarbeitung in der Medizin." In *Computer Magazin* 79, pp. 79ff.

Peterson, H.: "The Stockholm Country Medical Information System." In *Computer Information Systems in Health Care*, pp. 27ff. London: Sperry Univac, 1975.

Polli, George J.: "Medical Computing in the Small Clinic: Data Processing Alternatives and Their Economic Impact." Reprint of *Computers and Medicine, Special Report*. Chicago: American Medical Association, 1976.

Reichertz, P. L., J. R. Möhr, G. Holthoff, and E. Filsinger: *Struktur und Funktion der Allgemeinmedizinischen Praxis. Ergebnisse einer Analyse zur Untersuchung der Grundlagen für Computerunterstützung der Allgemeinmedizinischen Praxis. Projektzwischenbericht.* Köln, 1977.

Reichertz, P. L., G. von Gaertner-Holthoff, J. Möhr and B. Schwarz: *Struktur und Funktion der Allgemeinmedizinischen Praxis. Studie in Niedersachsen 1977.* Köln, 1978.

Reichertz, P. L., J. R. Möhr, B. Schwarz, A. Schlatter, G. von Gaertner-Holthoff, and E. Filsinger: "Evaluation of a Field Test of Computers for the Doctor's Office." In *Meth. Infor. Med.* 18(2):61ff., April 1979.

Sandscheper, Günter: "Kein Dr. med. Computer, aber sinnvolle Ablaufassistenz." In *Online-adlnachrichten*, No. 9, p. 647. Köln, 1978.

Schmidt, Herbert: *Das Sozialinformationssystem der Bundes-republik Deutschland. Sozialinnovation durch Informationstechnologie.* Eutin, 1977.

Schwarz, B., and P. L. Reichertz: "Motivationsuntersuchungen zur EDV-Einführung in der Arztpraxis – eine Delphi-Studie." Department für Biometrie und Medizinische Informatik, Medizinische Hochschule, Hannover, July 1978.

Van Egmond, J., P. F. De Vries Robbé, and A. H. Levy (eds.): "Information Systems for Patient Care." *Proceedings* of the IFIP Conference. Amsterdam: North-Holland, 1976.

Zimmerman, Joan: "Physician Utilization of Medical Records: Preliminary Determinations." *Med. Informatics* 3(1):27ff., 1978.

Zimmerman, Joan and Alan Rector: *Computers for the Physician's Office.* Forest Grove, 1978.

GERMAN-ENGLISH GLOSSARY OF SELECTED TERMS FOR ARCOS-CAPO

A

die ABRECHNUNG	Billing (procedure)
die ABRECHNUNGSDATEI	Billing — file
die AKTUALISIERUNG (Med. Dat.)	Update (med data)
die ANAMNESE	History (medical)
die ANWESENHEITSBESCHEINI-GUNG	Certificate of attendance
der ARZT	Physician
der ARZTBRIEF	Medican summary
das ARZT-COMPUTER-SYSTEM (ARCOS)	Physician's office computer system
die ARZTCOMPUTERANWENDUNG	Implementation of computers in physician's office
die ARZTPRAXIS	Medical practice

B

die BAUKASTENSTRUKTUR	Modular design (structure)
die BEFUNDE	Problems (findings)
die BESCHEINIGUNG	Certificate (form)
der BILDSCHIRM	(CRT) Screen
die BUCHHALTUNG	Accounting

D

die DATENÜBERMITTLUNG	Data transmission (communications)
die DATENVERARBEITUNG	Data processing
die DISKETTE	Diskette (floppy)
das DV-SYSTEM	Data processing system

E

die EDV (ELEKTRONISCHE DATENVERARBEITUNG)	EDP (electronic data processing)
die EINHEIT, PERIPHERIE	Peripheral unit
die ENTLASSUNG	Discharge (Patient)
der ENTSCHEIDUNGSTRÄGER	Decision maker
die ERFASSUNG, MEDIZINISCHE	Data entry (medical)

F

der FACHARZT   Specialist (medical)
die FACHGRUPPE   Specialty (group)

G

die GEBÜHRENORDNUNGSDATEI   File of (medical) service codes and
                                    fees
die GRUNDFUNKTIONEN   Basis applications

H

das HILFSMITTEL   Tool, *aid*

K

der KALENDER, TERMIN   Appointment schedule (book)
das KASSENREZEPT   Prescription paid by the insurance
                                    scheme
die KASSETTE   Magnetic cassette
das KRANKENBLATT   Medical record
  KRANKENKARTE
die KRANKENGESCHICHTE   Medical history
die KRANKENKASSE   Health insurance company
der KRANKENSCHEIN   (Health insurance) ID form
die KRANKENSCHEINMAHNUNG   Notice to submit ID form
die KV (KASSENÄRZTLICHE   German National health insurance plan
  VERSORGUNG)
die KV-ABRECHNUNG   Submission of claims (to NHIP)

L

der LEISTUNGSTAG   Date of service
die LEISTUNGSZIFFER   Service code
der LESESTIFT   Light pen

M

die MEDIKAMENTENVERORDNUNG Drug order
der MIKRORECHNER   Microcomputer
der MINI-RECHNER   Minicomputer

P

das PARAMEDIZINISCHE PERSONAL	Auxiliary staff (paraprofessionals)
die PATIENTEN-AUSWAHL	Patient selection (directory)
die PATIENTENANNAHME	Patient registration
die PATIENTENDATEI	Patient data (file)
die PRAXISGEGEBENHEITEN	Individual structure practice
der PRAXISINHABER	Head of medical practice
das PRAXISPERSONAL	Medical staff (personnel)
die PRIVATLIQUIDATION	Direct (private) invoice to patient (ex NHIP)
das PROGRAMMPAKET	Set of programs

R

das RECHENZENTRUM	Computer center

S

der SCHLÜSSEL	Code
die SOFTWAREWARTUNG	Software maintenance
der SPEICHER	Storage, memory
die STAMMDATEI	Basic-registration data
der STATUS PREASENS	Physical findings
die STORNO-MARKIERUNG	Cancellation (mark)

T

die TASTATUR	Keyboard
der TERMIN	Appointment (slot)
die TERMINPLANUNG	Scheduling (patient)
die TEXTAUTOMATENFUNK-TION	Word processing
die TEXTMASKE	Pre-formatted screen
die TRANSPARENTLISTE	Comparative list of drug prices

U

die UMSATZSTATISTIK	Utilization (statistics) — turnover

V

die VERSORGUNG, AMBULANTE	Ambulatory care
die VERSORGUNG, KASSENÄRZT- LICHE	(German) National health care plan
die VERWALTUNG, PATIENTEN	Patient administration
die VERWALTUNGSARBEIT	Administrative work
der VERWALTUNGSKOSTENSATZ	Administrative costs

W

die WARTELISTE	Waiting list
die WARTESCHLANGE	Waiting list (queue)
die WIRTSCHAFTLICHKEIT- SANALYSE	Analysis of economic effects
die WIRTSCHAFTLICHKEITSU- BERLEGUNG	Economic calculation

Z

das ZENTRALINSTITUT	Central Institute
der ZUGRIFF	Access (recall)

INDEX

A–2, 22
A–3, 22
Abacus, 3
Abbreviated codes, 128
A–B–C modules, 72
Academic medicine, 99
Access, 50
   forbidding, 116
   limited statutes, 114
   third party to medical records, 103
Accessed by the National Library of
   Medicine, viii
Accounting, viii, 65
   and billing, 143
Accounts, 148
Accounts payable, 77
Accounts receivable management, 77
ACTA scanner, 30
Action tree, 16
Actions on insurance policies, 120
Adaptation and diversity, 22
Adding machine, 6, 7
Administrative work in doctor's practice, 174
Admission–discharge–transfer, 129
Admission policies, medical schools, 100
Admitting office, 128
Advanced clinical information system, 88
Advanced computer system in laboratory,
   132
Advancing electronic technology, 130
Adverse drug reactions, ix
Age of computers, 2
Aggregate of computer programs, 101
Algebraic family, 50
ALGOL, 50
Algorithm, 2, 3, 50
Algorithmic machines, 18
Algorithms, 5, 16
Alpha micro (am100), 151
Alphanumeric keyboard, 133
Ambulatory treatment, 172, 176

American Medical Association, 104
American Nurses Association code, 104
American Psychiatric Association, 112
American Society of Internal Medicine, 76
Amount of disc storage, 77
Amount of memory, 77
Analog computer(s), 22, 51
Analytic machine, 8, 9
Analytic reconstruction, 46
Analyzers to computers, 132
APA, 112
Apple II, 75
Application of computers to medical prac-
   tice, 75
Application specifications, 79
Appointment scheduling, 65, 77
Appointment slots, 71
Appointments, 69
Arcos, 179
Arcos commands, 180
Artificial intelligence, 14, 17
Artificial medical memory, 95
Assault on privacy, 120
Attorney-client relationship, 103
Attorney recommendations, 86
Audible codes, 51
Australia, computer in medical practice, 141
Authorization, consent, 109
Authorization program, 92
Autoanalyzers, 132
Automated decoding, 92
Automated encoding, 91
Automatic analyzer(s), 131, 132
Automatic computer, 9
Automatic control in medicine, 20
Automatic monitoring of patient, 139
Automatic multitest laboratories, 39
Automatic phototypesetting, 137
Automatic programming, 18
Automation, 20, 44, 76
Availability of service, 84

Babbage's analytical engine, 10
Babbage's difference engine, 11
BACAIC, 22
Bach reconstruction, 46
Back up Installations, 81
Bank, clinical experience, 93
Bank, knowledge, 94
BASIC, 22
Basic machine language, 22
Batch processing, 127
Batch system, 26
Bayes strategy, 21
Bayes theorem, 16
Bayesian diagnosis, 21
Bedside, and computer, 139
Behavioral interactions, 173
Benefits in business efficiency, 76
Billing, viii, 65, 151
    and accounting, 69
    and scheduling, 93
Billing documents, 71
Binary digits, 22
Binary numbers, 51
Biological data, 15
Biology, 20
Biomedical research bank, 98
Biopsychosocial health, 22, 49
Biosocial development, 21
Birth certificates, 107
Bit, 51
Bits, 22
Bits of information, 18
Black box, 75
Blanket authorizations, 112
Block directory, 98
Blue sky, 152
Body scanner, 46
Bookkeeping, 7
Boolian algebra, 51
Breast cancer, 43
British India, 37
Business accounting, 77
Business and personal tax, 143
Business office, 125
Buy a comprehensive system, 87
Buying a computer, 76
Buzz words, 75
Byte, 51

Calculating machine(s), 7, 11
Calculator, 3
Calculus of probabilities, 7
Call ins, 71
Canada, health care system, 129
Canadian Medical Association, 182
Cancer cartography, 39
Cancer, geographic pathology of, 38
Cancer research, 38
Cancer in the United States, 36
Candor, 105
Capacity of human memory, 89
Capital-intensive computer, 125
Capitation fees, 169
Cartesian coordinates, 37
Cartography, 36
Case history bank, 92
Case summaries, 93
Cathode ray tube, 51
Cathode ray tube (CRT) console, 30
CCU (coronary care units), 38
Central register, 127
Certificates, birth and death, 107
Character of information, 51
Character of patients, 104
Characterization of human tumors, 49
Charges, 77
Check ups, 71
Chemical abstracts, 15
Child neglect and abuse, 107
Children, 108
Civilized man's most valued right, 120
Classification of medical terms, 97
Client of the care service, 127
Clients of government health services, 111
Client's right to privacy, 104
Clinic managers, 68
Clinical data, 93
Clinical experience bank, 93
Clinical services rendered, 93
Clinical signs, arcs, 97
Clinics, outpatient, 129
Cloth manufacturing, 8
Cluster analysis, 16
Cluster of arcs, 97
COBOL, 22, 27
Code(s), 2, 146
    abbreviated, 91, 128
    American nurses, 104

Code of Hammurabi, 2
Coded data, 52
Cognitive cascade of arcs, 96
Cognitive mental process, 89
Collection notices, 77
Colored screens, 128
Combinatorial games, 28
Common binary language, 22
Common law right of inspection, 115
Communicable diseases, 107
Communication, 90, 103
    codes, 13, 22
    with the computer, 152
    devices, 66
    interdisciplinary, 182
    interhuman, 94
    links, 24, 28
    medical, 89
    of Scientific Information by S. B. Day,
        48
Communications, datenubermittlung, 184
Communications made to a doctor, 120
Community, 30
Companion To The Life Sciences, 48
Complete history, 72
Comprehensive directories, 127
Computable knowledge, 89
Computable medical knowledge, 99
Computer(s), 51, 66, 141, 151
    bedside, and medical record, 139
    in biology, 39
    capital-intensive, 125
    in diagnosis, 21
    and disorganized practice, 78
    in doctor's office, 172
    for doctor's practices, 173
    effectiveness of, 172
    filing, 127
    health records, and patient rights, 119
    hybrid, 22
    in hospitals, 65, 125
    and instrumentation, 138
    large scale systems, viii
    legal aspects of, ix
    legislation, ix
    in medical practice, vii
    and medicine, 87
    for physicians, vii
    private practice, 65

Computer(s) (continued)
    smallness and cheapness, 125
    types of, 22
    United Kingdom experience, 157
    for word processing, 137
Computer age, 3
Computer-aided records, 71
Computer-aided systems, 65
Computer analyses, 158
Computer application in hospitals, 125
Computer basics, 75
Computer capability, 14
Computer cartography, 31, 36, 49
    of cancer data, 38, 49
    and disease, 37
Computer centers, 112
    policy, 113
Computer/communications technology, 65,
    66, 73
Computer development, vii
Computer display of cancer data, 49
Computer driven typewriter, 128
Computer generations, 12, 24
Computer graphic systems, 30
Computer information, 37
Computer language, 50, 52
Computer marketplace, 76
Computer medicine, 39, 46
Computer memory, 71
Computer methodologies, 1
Computer modelling and cancer data,
    49
Computer modelling of data, 49
Computer operation, 68
Computer programs, 25
Computer science, 75
Computer skills, 75
Computer stored ambulatory rec. system,
    65
Computer support of medicine, 89
Computer systems, 23, 65
Computer technology, 24, 100
Computer terminals, 90
Computer testing, 73
Computerization, 65
    of medical records, 103
    of patient scheduling, 69
    in private practice, 68

Computerized environmental data, 49
Computerized information system, 66
Computerized mapping of disease, 31, 49
Computerized medical records, 110
Computerized record(s), 128, 132
Computerized systems, reliability, 140
Computerized task, 77
Concept of cancer, 49
Concept of feedback, 72
Concept of specialization, 88
Concept of zero, 1
Concepts, 89
    of molecular structure, 18
Confidences, 104
Confidentiality, 73, 102
    in a computer network, 149
    legal concepts of, 103
Congressional privacy commission, 112
Consent, 109
    minors, 113
Console, 51
Constitutional right of privacy, 103
Contagious and dangerous diseases, 107
Continuity of records, 116
Contract negotiation, 85, 87
Contracts, 85
Control equipment, 9
Control management information systems,
    15
Control systems, 19
Controlling knowledge, 88
Conversational mode, 128
Coping with unpredictable factors, 71
Core memory, 51
Coroner, 107
Correct information, 102
Correcting errors, 117
COSTAR, 65
Cost and time expenditure, 76
Cost containment, 126
Cost of additional compilers, 81
Cost of leasing, 148
Cost of processing charges, 76
Cost/benefit study, 76
Cost-efficient systems, 67
Counting frame, 3
Court's interest, 105
Courts, 105
    discretion, 109

Criminally inflicted injuries, 107
Criteria for selection of computer, 75
Cross referencing, 91
CRT, 51
    format displays, 79
    screen, 137
    CRT terminal, 137
Culture shock, 170
Cumulative aide-memoire, 72
Cumulative patient profiles, 69
Current medications, 72
Custodian, 109
Cybernetics, 17, 19
Cybernex (A), 154

Daily transactions, 77
Data, 9, 12, 52
    in Canada, 126
    in Europe, 126
    guidelines for use of aggregate in re-
        search, 119
    quantity of, 157
    in U.S.A., 126
Data analysis, 13
Data bank/patient, 90
Data banks, 14, 92
    in a free society, 120
Data base, 52
Data bases via a modem, ix
Data decay, 158
Data flow, 174
Data reduction, 37
Data security, 14
Data source, 92
Data systems, public notice of, 119
Death certificates, 107
Debit and credit analysis, 143
DEC, 66
Decision functions, 89
Decision-making powers, 19
Decision, physician of, 152
Decision under risk, 21
Decisions, 19
Define specifications, 79
Defining requirements, 78
Defining the practice needs, 87
Definition arc, 97
Demographic data, 72
Deposit medical knowledge, 95

Design principles, 65, 72
Design of medical information systems, 66
Design and writing of group computer programs, 144
Developing an education-computer, 87
Developing an expertise, 75
Developing sea power, 7
Development of societies, 4
Diagnosis/therapy, 88
Diagnostic calculations, 39
Diagnostic categories, 164
Diagnostic codes, 73
Diagnostic files, 94
Diagnostic study arcs, 97
Difference engine, 9
Digital computers, 17, 22, 51
Digital Equipment Corporation, 66
Digital processors, 51
Directed graph(s), 28, 30
Directories, comprehensive, 127
Discharges, 129
Disclosure
    of confidential information, 122
    to family members, 113
    to an insurance company, 105
    of intimate details, 106
    to other health providers, 113
    to a spouse, 105
Discriminant analysis, 16
Disease description, 46
Disk drives, 73
Display, 51
Display maps, 38
Distribution of disease agent, 34
District attorney, 107
Doctor, communications made to, 120
Doctor's maximum effort, 69
Doctor's office, 151
Doctor's practice, 174
Doctor-patient relationship, 103
    improved relationship, 116
Doctors, 65
    in the Federal Republic of Germany
        (1978), 173
Documentation, 25
    of transactions, 77
Down time experience, 80
Down time response, 84
Drop in, 71

Drug interactions, ix
Drug usage, 170

Earth Resources Technology Satellite
    (LANDSAT I), 37
Ecologic factors, evaluation of, 34
EDP, 52
EDP system, 172
Education, 82
    of the practitioner, 89
EDVAC, 12
Effectiveness of computers, 172
Eight bit bytes, 51
Electronic computational device, 22
Electronic computers, 11
Electronic computing machines, 20
Electronic data processing for medical
    office, 75
Electronic data processing machines 52
Electronic data processing machines, 52
Electronic data processing systems, 44
Emergency information, 72
Enhanced patient care, vii
ENIAC, 11
Epidemiologic arcs, 97
Equipment installation, 73
Erroneous identification, 127
Errors, correcting, 117
Established patients, 77
Ethics, 103
Evaluating needs, 76
Evaluation, 98
Everyday work of the practice, 179
Evolution of computers, 9
Evolutions of systems, 1
Examination, 146
Exceptions to confidentiality, 107
Existing law of medical privacy, 103
Expandable family of computers, 84
Expansion of system, 78
Expectations from a computer, 76
Expected constraints by computers, 177
Expected improvements by computers, 177
Experimental hypotheses, 89
Extended case summary, 93

Fact, 96
Factor analysis, 16
Factoring in intangibles, 76

Family file, 145
Family master record files, 143
Family members, disclosure, 113
Family practice, 125
Feasible medical office computer system, 75
Federal Republic of Germany, health care, 172
Feedback of information, 176
Feedback mechanism, 11
Fidelity of verbalization, 90
File(s), 13, 69
    family, 145
Financial module, 69, 71
Findings, 98
Five-year costs, 86
Five-year operating plan, 78
Floating pool, nurses, 127
Floppy disc, 161
Forbidding access, 116
Formal knowledge, 101
FORTRAN, 22, 25, 50
Freedom of information, 102
Furnish any or all information on request, 112
Future technology, 5

Game playing, 18
Gap between knowledge and care, 88
General interest magazines, 75
General medical practice, 141
General medical scheme insurers, 173
General practitioner, 157
General-purpose computer, 12
General release forms, 109
General risk index, 158
Genetic arcs, 97
Geographic data, 36
Geographic pathology of disease, 49
Georgia free consent experiment, 122
German Doctor's Association, 181
German-English glossary, 184
German health system, 172
Glossary, German-English, 184
Goal tree, 16
Government-sponsored projects, Germany, 175
Graphics, 14
    technology, 30
Group practice, 71

Growth of medical knowledge, 88
Guidelines for use of aggregate data in research, 119

Handling information, 14
Handling of texts, 181
Hardware, 22, 25, 52, 73
Hardware configuration, 79
Hardware expansion capability, 84
Hardware of implemented doctor's office, 175
Hardware information, 79
Hardware maintenance, 80
Hardware for mumps, 181
Hardware requirements, 142
Hardware spectrum, 175
Harvard Mark I, 11
Health care delivery system, 125
Health care professionals, 66
Health care providers, 103
Health care system of Canada, 129
Health communications, 48, 90
Health Communications and Biopsychosocial Health, vii
Health data, 31
Health delivery network, 35
Health informatics, 1, 19, 65
Health insurance coverage in F. R. of Germany, 173
Health network, 30
Health providers, disclosure to, 113
Health specialist, 30
Hew medical malpractice commission, 115
Hierarchical values, 2
High-level languages, 25
Hippocratic oath, 104
Histories and physicals, 77
History, 146
Hospital information system, 134
Hospital to release information, 109
Hospital's budget, 129
Hospitals, scene in, 128
Human brain, 12
Human information processing, 14
Human knowledge, 13
Human memory, 13, 88

IBM 704 computer, 25
Ideas, 89
Image reconstruction (IRC), 45
Implementing care, 104
Implied consent, 109
Improved efficiency, 77
Improved medical records, 77
Improvement in clinical performance, 170
Increased patient information, 116
Indian system of numerals, 5
Individuals and society, 105
Industrial organization, 8
Industry jargon, 75
Indus Valley civilizations, 4
Inexpensive microcomputers, viii
Infinite whole, 3
Information, 9, 28
    carbon copy to patients, 116
    chemical, 15
    communicated to physician, 105
    communication, 46
    content of clinical decisions, 89
    deficit in medicine, 88
    display, 90
    about drugs, 158
    in electronics, 15
    expression of, 18
    furnish on request, 112
    general, 15
    injudicious disclosure of, 104
    input, 19
    medical, 88
    medical, releasing, 103
    measuring, 20
    nursing stations, 129
    on space, 15
    overload, 36
    processing psychology, 18
    protection of, 102
    retrieval, 15
    specifics, 112
    storage, 17
    system, patient, 127
Information systems, vii, 66, 102
    transfer, 38
    usage, 4
Informational privacy of the individual, 106
Injudicious disclosure of information, 104
Inpatient care, 126

Input, 13, 19
Input/output, 52
    devices, 22
Inquirer, 49
Inquiring system, 49
Inquiry, 50
Installation of computer, 73
Instructive articles on computers, 75
Instrumentation, and computers,
    138
Insurance claim forms, 77
Insurance coverage, 126
Int. Fndtion. Biosoc. Dev. & Hum. Health,
    48
Intangible benefits, 86
Integral calculus, 6
Integrated data banks, 92
Integrated file of data, 52
Integrated societies, 2
Integrity of medical record, 117
Intelligent terminal, 131
Interacting sub-systems, 131
Interactive computer graphics, 30
Interactive graphics, 14
Interdisciplinary communication, 182
Interface, man-machine, 90
Interference, unwarranted state, 118
Interhuman communication, 94
International Business Machines Corpora-
    tion (IBM), 11
International comparison, 182
Introduction to computers, 75
Invalidity of blanket surgical consent,
    110
Invasions of privacy, 106
I/O, 52
Isorithms, 35
Isotope scanners, 44
Item no., 146
Iterative reconstruction, 46

Jacquard attachment, 9
Jacquard's machine, 9
Judicial process, 108

Kaiser-Permanente system, 65
Keyboard, 12
Keyboard-equipped video terminal, 132
Keypunch, 52

Knowledge, 7, 17, 88, 104
  acousticophonetic, 18
  common sense, 18
  heuristic, 18
  of transfers and discharges, 129
  sources of, 18
  well organized, 66
  yielding total information, 92
Knowledge bank, 94
Knowledge-based systems, 14
Knowledge engineering, 14, 17
Knowledge management, 19
Krankenkassen, 173

Laboratories, 44
Laboratory, 131
  reports, 72
Language, 13, 75
  of mathematics, 2
  of numbers, 4
Language, supported by system, 81
Laser beam printer, 137
Late physician, 69
Law, 102
  and ethics, 103
  and medical records, 102
Leakage from medical records system,
  109
Learning system, 26
Legal aspects of computers, ix
  of confidentiality, 103
  of privacy, 103
Legal duty of physicians, 104
Legal obligation, 108
Legality of release form, 113
Letter by letter match, 91
Lex talionis, 2
Lexical entry, 91
Lexicon, 18, 91
Light pen, 51, 128
Likelihood of being hoodwinked, 76
Limitations of system, 84
Limited practice, 76
List of hospitalizations, 72
Litigation, ix
Location, dates, cost per education, 82
Logarithmic tables, 6
Logarithms, 5
Logic, 52

Machine era, 50
Machine-independent languages, 22
Machine intelligence, 16
Machine language, 22
Machine logic, 52
Machine steps, 9
Machine vision, 18
Magnetic tape, 12
Malpractice cases, 108
Man and computer, 37
Man-computer systems, 90
Man-machine interface, 90
Man-machine system, 89
Manchester university, 162
Mandatory disclosures, 107
Manual filing, 127
Manual operations, 68
Manual systems in doctor's offices, viii
Manufacturer, 83
Mapping of diseases, 37, 39
Mapping of total cancer, 39
Maps, 31, 35
Marginal punched cards, 39
Mass storage, 66
Mass. Gen. Hosp. Utility Multi-Pro. Syst., 71
Master file, 77
Mathematical functions, 28
Mayo Clinic System, 65
Mechanical slaves, 21
Medical audit, 72
Medical communication, 21, 89
Medical cybernetics, 21
Medical decision making, 39
Medical diagnosis, 16, 39
Medical examiner, 107
Medical information, 21
  minors, 113
Medical information systems, vii, 66, 73,
  141
Medical insurance organizations, 126
Medical knowledge, 88
Medical knowledge bank, 90
Medical lexicon, 94
Medical message, 94
Medical practice, 67
Medical privacy, 102
Medical profession, 141
Medical professionals, 65
  and health insurance, 173

Medical record processing, 39
Medical record storage system, 144
Medical records, 77, 102, 106, 144, 147
  and bedside, 139
  and the law, 102
  du Pont, 112
  never alter, 117
  ownership of, 114
  possession of, 114
Medical records module, 69, 71
Medical recording, viii
Medical recording issue, 72
Medical-related technology, VII
Medical school curriculum, 99
Medical storage data, 141
Medical terms, 101
Medical text, 91
Medical training, 88
Medical university generator, 71
Medical users, 67
Medical/health care packages, 66
Mental health computer file, 111
Medical/health information network, 47
Medication orders, 130
Memorizable material, 100
Memory, 13, 88
Menu display, 153
Menu screen, 164
Menus, 66
Message, 98
Method for providing solution, 50
Methods of communication, 38
Minicomputer(s), viii, 125, 135
Microcomputer, 125, 158
Microfiche, 128
Microfilm/microfiche, 137
Microprocessors, 22
Micro-scanner, evolution of, 44
Minors, 113
Model, 98
Modelling, 16
Modelling systems, 15
Modems, 156
  for adverse drug actions, ix
  for new pharmaceuticals, ix
  for post-graduate medical education, ix
Modern computer, 8
Modern statistical theory, 4
Modular approach, 67

Modular medical information system, 67
Molecular models, 45
Monitoring drug usage, 170
Monitoring progress, 72
Monitoring quality of care, 116
Monthly tasks, 77
MUG, 71
Multiphasic screening program, 39
Multiphasing screening, 72
Multiple billing, 126
MUMPS, 71, 180
MYCIN, 19

Napier's bones, 7
Nation's health service, 30
  British, 158
Natural language communication, 90
Need to know basis, 119
Needs of clinic management, 73
Nerve networks, 20
Network, 27
  analysis, 28
  designs, 30
  synthesis, 27, 28
    application, 27
New knowledge, 36
New patients, 77
New pharmaceuticals, ix
New technologies, 157
Nightmare of medical practice solved, 69
No disclosures, 113
Nodal center, 30
Nodes, 95
Non-believer role, vii
Nuclear medicine, 30
Number and size language, 1
Numbers, 30
  in navigation, 4
  information usage, 1
Numeric or nonnumeric data, 52
Nurse-client relationship, 104
Nurse's time, 130
Nurses, 130
Nursing care payroll, 129
Nursing station, 129
  enter information, 129

OFMs, 83
Office computerization, 66
Office systems, viii
OHIP, 156
Online commands, 25
On-line inquiry, 72
Online programming language, 25
On-line typewriters, 128
Ontario health insurance plan, 153
Open-ended authorizations, 112
Operations research, 16
Operative and consultation reports, 77
Optional disclosure, 109
OR, 16
Ordinary graph, 30
Organized cognitive matrix, 95
OSHA, 112
Outpatient clinics, 129
Output, 13, 19
Outside equipment manufacturers, 83
Ownership of medical records, 114

Paper, total displacement of, 170
Paralanguage, 90
    of medicine, 90
Partnership, 71
Past clinical experience, 88
Past medical history, 101
Patient and office management, 66
Patient challenge, 117
Patient data bank, 90
Patient education, 65
Patient education programs, 76
Patient files, 93
Patient follow up, 72
Patient history files, 143
Patient identifiers, 93
Patient information system, 127
Patient management, 147
Patient privacy, ix
Patient profile structure, 147
Patient records, 65, 72
Patient registration, viii
    files, 73
Patient scheduling, viii
Patients, 77
Patient to show good cause, 114
Patient/physician relationships, ix
Patient-related information, 89

Patient's right to their own medical records, 123
Pattern concept, 8
Pattern-making technology, 9
Patterns of communication, 28
Pattern vocabulary, 18
Payroll, 77, 126
Peer review, 72
    programs, 89
Performance data, 179
Peripherals, 84
Personal-data-keeping systems, 102
Personal privacy in the computer age, 121
Personal privacy in an information society, 122
Personnel, 81
Pertinent clinical experience, 101
Pertinent information for clinician, 89
PET, 75
Pharmacology, 30
Physical examinations, 72
Physician, 75
    costs, 129
    education, ix
    orientated periodicals, 76
Physician's office systems, 65
Physician/institution identifiers, 93
Physician/patient relationship, ix
Physicians, primer on computers, 156
Physicians, records and knowledge, 92
Physicians records and knowledge, 92
Pixels, 37
PL/1, 22, 26
Plans, 146
Policy, computer centers, 113
Possession of record, 114
Post-graduate medical education, ix
Postindustrial society, 15, 50
PRAKTICE, 88, 92, 93, 96
    medicine, VII
Practitioner-patient relationship, 102
Preparing information on charges, 71
Preprogramming machines, 11
Priest-penitent relationship, 103
Primary service, 182
Principle of ethics, 104
Principles of computer, 19
PRINT, 22
Printed medical records, 71

Printed reports, 66
Printing, laser beam, 138
Privacy, 73
    and freedom, 106
    legal concepts of, 103
Privacy Act 1974, 115
Private interest of patient, 110
Privilege, 103
    by statute, 105
    rule of evidence, 103
Privilege doctrine, 105
Probability occurrence, 21
Problem name, 146
Problem-oriented medical information system, 65
Problem-solving literature, 16
Problems of interfacing, 177
Procedure, 98
Productivity profiles on each physician, 77
Professional Standards review organization, 108
Profit of computerization, 140
Program, 52
Program budgeting, 127
Programmer, experienced, 151
Programming language(s), 22, 24, 73, 81
Programming technology, 24
Programming theory, 24
Progress notes, 72, 145, 149
Progress of patient's illness, 72
Projects agency (ARPA), 34
PROMIS, 65
Promise of secrecy, 105
Promote full disclosure, to, 104
Protecting information, 102
Provider policy, 117
Pseudo-science, 21
PSRO, 118
Public concern, 110
Public health and diseases, 107
Public health statistics, 31
Public notice of all data systems, 119
Public policy, 102
Public reporting statutes, 107
Punched cards, 9, 12
    use of, 11
Purchase of a computer, 87
Purchaser-basic knowledge, 76
Pursuit of health, 105

Quality of care, ix
Quality of consent, 113
Quality of health care, ix
Quality of medical services, 71
Quality of records, 118
Quantitative discriminators, 17
Quasi-systems, 50

Radiology, 131
Radiology systems, 136
Random access, 50
Real life situations, and computer, 141
Real-time systems, 128
Real world, 19
Receipts, 77
Recommendations, privacy commission, 112
Reconstructed tomography, 45
Record keeping, 102
Record, possession, 114
References, 98
Referral letters, 77
Regular appointments, 71
Regulating systems, 22
Related clinical experiences, 89
Related formal medical knowledge, 89
Relationship
    client-attorney, 103
    doctor-patient, 103
    priest-penitent, 103
Release forms, 112
Releasing medical information, 103
Reliability of computerized systems, 140
Relicensing, 89
Reports to public agencies, 109
Reputations of manufacturer, 83
Request for proposal, 78
Requirements to make available certain records, 123
Rescheduling of patient, 69
Research, guidelines for use of aggregate data, 119
RFP, 78
Right of privacy, 106
Right to be let alone, 103
Robots, 18
Rush, 26

Salaries of personnel, 76
Scheduling patients in waves, 71
Schemes of insurance, 126
Science and technology, 5
Science literacy, 2
Screens, colored, 128
Search, 91
Secret, presumption of, 103
Secretarial acceptance, 152
Selection criteria, 75
    (software), 85
Selection of alpha micro, 154
Self-responsibility of patient, 176
Semantic content, 90
Sensor instruments, 139
Serial access, 50
Servo systems, 20
Shedding device, 9
Shift differentials, 126
Shipping lanes, 4
Size language, 2
Sloan Kettering Institute for Cancer Re-
    search, 46
Small home computer, 75
Smooth flow of patients, 69
Social Darwinism, 21
Society, 102
    vs. technology, 14
Software, 25, 52, 143
Software compatibility in upgrades, 84
Software conversion, 84
Software definition, 81
Software selection maintenance, 85
Solo practice, 71
Soviet Union, 20
Space satellites, 36
Space vehicles, 3
Spatial conceptualizations, 38
Spatial data, 38
Specific protections of privacy, 106
Specifics of information, 112
Staff training, 73
Staff wages, 148
Standard teletypewriters, 132
State and federal laws, 102
State interference, unwarranted, 118
State medical licensing boards, 115
State of Georgia-information, 110
Statements, 77

Statistical reporting, 77
Statutes regarding physicians, 103
Statutory adoption of privilege, 105
Steam power, 8
Storage capacity, viii
Storage space, 90
Stored data, 73
Student and learning, 95
Substitute equipment, 84
Sunshine Acts, 102
Sunya, 3
Supreme Court, U.S., 103
Surnames, 127
Sweden, ix
Symbol data capture, 14
Symbolic problem solving, 18
Symbols, 3, 17
Synopsis, 93
Syntax, 18, 90
    of ideal language, 6
System conversion, 73
System software support, 73, 84
System in action, 85
System of communication, 4
Systems approach, 50
Systems era, 50
Systems in practice, viii
Systems science, 50
Systems theory, 50

Tabulating machine company, 11
Tandy TRS 80, 171
Tape systems, 149
Tax deductions, 76
Teach computer to understand, 90
Technocon, 65
Technocracies, 5
Technological improvements, 8
Technology, 66
    and power, 7
    of a modern society, 149
    video terminal, 131
Telephone links, 156
Teletype, 17
Telling of impending death, 110
Terminal, 51, 68
Terminal keyboard, 26
Terminals, 24
Terms for arcos-capo, 184

Territorial behavior of animals, 106
Text editors, 137
Textbooks, 88
Theories, 89
Theory of meaning, 90
Therapeutic patterns, 72
Therapy arcs, 97
Thinking, 17
Thinking "in numbers", 38
Thinking process and ideas, 89
Thinking robots, 21
Third party access to medical records,
    103
Third party billing, 71
Time management module, 69
Time-related statistics, 94
Time sharing, viii
Time-sharing systems, 125
Timetables for physicians, 71
Tin mikes, 21
To be free of peeping, snooping, 103
Total clinic system for group practice, 67
Total displacement of paper, 170
Trade routes, 5
Tradition and ethics of medicine, viii
Traditional method of learning, 89
Transcultural communications, 5
Transfer of patient data, viii
Treatment, 146
TRS 80, 75
Trust, 104
Truth, 105
Tumor-cell kinetics, 36
Turnkey system, 67
Tutorial learning, 95
Types of cancer, 39
Types of information, 89
Typewriter, computer driven, 128
Typewriter keyboard, 51
Typhoid in towns, 37

Uganda Africans, 31
Uncoded data, 52

Unified record, 129
Unit of information, 51
United States based packages, 136
UNIVAC I, 12
Universal language, 25
Universal machine, 17
Unwarranted state interference, 118
Urban centers, 30
U.S. population density, 42
User growth rate, 84
User oriented systems, 68

VDTs, 66
VDU capacity, 142
Vendor, 82
Vendor selection, 83, 87
Vendors, 78
Verbalize ideas, 89
Video display units, 72
Video terminal technology, 131
Video terminals, 128
Vishnevskiy Institute, 21
Visual images, 30
Vital statistics, 107
Volume of data, 126
Volume of medical information,
    88

Warning to avert danger, 108
Warranties, 86
Wave Approach, 71
What is a Machine?, 17
Wills, 120
Writing a request for a proposal, 87
Writing programs, 76

X-ray CAT scanner, 45
X-ray photography, 44
X-ray reports, 72
X-rays diagnosis, 45

Zero, 3
Zero-based budgeting, 127